CW00880279

because, seriously
who has time?

# 2 WEEKS
# TO FEELING
# GREAT

gabriela peacock

An Hachette UK Company
www.hachette.co.uk

First published in Great Britain in 2021 by
Kyle Books, an imprint of
Octopus Publishing Group Limited
Carmelite House
50 Victoria Embankment
London EC4Y 0DZ
www.kylebooks.co.uk

ISBN: 978 0 85783 963 3

Distributed in the US by Hachette Book Group,
1290 Avenue of the Americas,
4th and 5th Floors, New York, NY 10104

Distributed in Canada by Canadian Manda Group,
664 Annette St., Toronto, Ontario,
Canada M6S 2C8

Publisher: Jo Copestick
Editorial Director: Judith Hannam
Writer: Clare Bennett
Senior Commissioning Editor: Louise McKeever
Design: Nikki Dupin at Studio Nic&Lou
Copy-editor: Sophie Elletson
Food photography: Kate Whitaker
Food stylist: India Whiley-Morton
Lifestyle photography: Kate Martin
Lifestyle photography assistant: Ben Ottewell
Production: Lisa Pinnell

A Cataloguing in Publication record for this title is
available from the British Library.

Printed and bound in Italy.

10 9 8 7 6 5 4 3 2 1

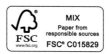

# Gabriela Peacock

Gabriela Peacock qualified as a Nutritional Therapist with BSc (Hons) in Health
Science from the University of Westminster and a diploma in Naturopathic
Nutrition, going on to set up her first clinic in Belgravia in 2012.

Gabriela's work focuses on achieving optimum health through a realistic approach
to modern life. In 2016, she founded GP Nutrition, launching her own range of
specialised supplement programmes. Gabriela lives in West London with her
husband and three children.

# contents

# introduction

I once lived on green beans. That was, quite literally, all I ate. I was 16, starting out as a model and was told to eat nothing but green beans to lose weight (don't get me wrong, I love green beans; they're high in vitamin C and magnesium... but, er, hello..?). I now eat every three to four hours – in fact, when I got married, my orthodontist ticked me off for constantly taking out my braces to have my snacks. Times have radically changed.

After a 15-year career as a model, what I realised when studying nutrition at university in London is that knowledge is power. Funnily enough – and I hope you're sitting down for this – it turns out that starving yourself on only green beans is not a healthy, safe way to lose weight. Nine years' studying and two degrees later, I am still amazed at how clever the body is, having seen first-hand in my clinic how even adding one supplement to your diet can quickly change the way you feel.

There is so much information on weight loss and nutrition now. Everyone has an opinion on diets, food and supplements – but inevitably, that comes with judgement. If you're not reaching your target weight, it's your fault. If you haven't signed up for every HIIT class at the gym, you're lazy. There are tons of guides on how to manage weight and be healthy, but very few have a realistic approach for people with real lives.

What I know through years of experience is that you don't have to make huge changes to reach your goals. We're all so busy in this day and age – travelling, working and raising children – that we need to find ways to feel fantastic that are simple and achievable, which is why this book is full of my easy tricks and tips. You can make improvements without feeling stressed or overwhelmed and take it as far as you want. All roads lead to feeling better than ever before. The bottom line is, you don't have to be perfect throughout your journey and I have no inclination to judge anyone for their choices. I am a nutritionist, and I quite regularly eat last night's takeaway curry for breakfast (okay, with quinoa rather than white rice, but still) because I'm probably tired, possibly a little bit hungover and definitely can't be bothered to make something fresh while my two youngest are throwing bits of scrambled eggs at each other.

My aim with this book is to educate you so that you understand how your body works as an interconnected system and the ways to make it function at its highest level. Once you have that knowledge, you can dip in and out of these pages, depending on what you need at any particular time – whether you're exhausted after Christmas, going through a bad sleeping phase or have had one too many rosé lunches over the summer. I encourage you to live life and have fun. You don't have to be hysterical about your health in order to feel great. Life really is too short.

# A note on the magic of supplements

To say I'm obsessed with supplements is an understatement. These concentrated forms of goodness may come in tiny quantities, but they have a potent and targeted biochemical effect within the body. They are not designed to replace healthy food but to *supplement* it; together they become a power couple of epic proportions.

People often ask me why they need supplements if their diet is healthy. The influences of stress, alcohol, late nights, not enough exercise, pollution and that expensive anti-wrinkle cream that is actually full of parabens, are daily challenges. Along with all the normal processes within the body that are draining it of nutrients, these kinds of external factors all contribute to the body having to redirect the nutrients it needs to flourish to prioritise what it considers to be harmful. And if it's any consolation, I am yet to meet a single patient who doesn't present with any kind of deficiency. To make this a whole lot simpler, I will be including lists of my favourite nutrient supplements, along with the food and lifestyle recommendations, at the end of every chapter. I encourage you to try them and see what works for you – or at the very least, start with a good-quality multi-nutrient.

## GENERAL RULES FOR CHOOSING SUPPLEMENTS

- **POTENCY** – check the percentage of the nutrient in the daily recommended intake. It should be high – anything from about 80 per cent upwards. Low amounts indicate it has been cheaply made and will have a limited effect.

- **BIOAVAILABILITY** – good brands will choose forms of nutrients that are more easily absorbed by the body. Plus, they often combine them with other substances to maximise this effect.

- **CONVENIENCE** – there are many ways to take supplements – pill form, capsules, powder, drinks. Choose the one that suits you and will encourage you to keep taking them.

My supplement fixation resulted in me creating my very own range. OBVIOUSLY they tick all the boxes I have just described, plus they are super goal-focused and provide support for the topics we'll be talking about. It's such a coincidence, they are all listed as scannable codes on page 204... What could be easier?

# 1/

# GP principles *for* healthy weight loss

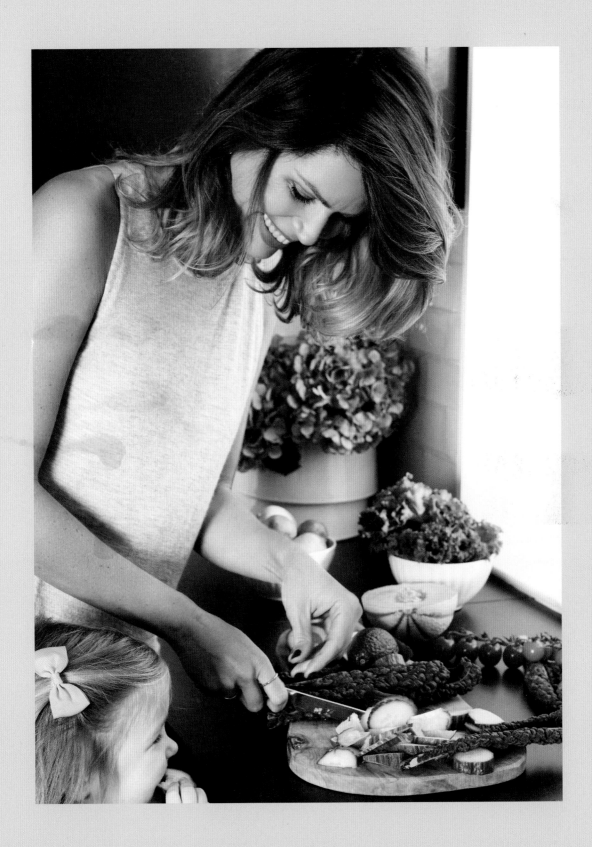

*You're here...* Exciting. Feeling thinner yet? Okay, so there's more to weight loss and feeling great than just buying a book – but making the decision to want to feel better and be healthier is the first big step. Some people find the thought of making changes to their diet and lifestyle daunting, but I can assure you that it's far less of an ordeal than you might think. Be kind to yourself and remember that I am here to guide you. No one is going to starve or be made to cry. You deserve to feel fantastic. Let's get started.

# why weight matters

The concept of weight loss is much more complicated than simply stripping the body of fat, as many diets suggest. The fact is the human body needs fat – not too little and not too much. Fat plays an important role in protecting, insulating and storing energy, so it's not just a question of shedding pounds, but about maximising overall health.

While no one should obsess over their weight, it's critical not to ignore being overweight. Weight loss is not just about getting slimmer now, but about safeguarding your health. No one should be ashamed of wanting to look their best, but becoming thin enough to wrestle your way into a pair of skinny jeans should not be the only goal. In addition, what someone might deem a target weight may not actually be appropriate for their height.

So many of us step onto the scales and believe that the number we see is indicative of how fat we are. That is simply not true, as body weight depends on many different factors, including muscle mass, bone density and fluid levels, as well as fat (adipose tissue). Improving exercise regimes inevitably increases muscle tone. While this will make our body mass heavier, more muscle will also help regulate how fast and efficiently food is processed and used. This is one of the reasons I don't care for scales. Becoming fixated with the results on a weighing device is destructive and should never be the deciding factor in how we feel about our bodies.

The reality is that being overweight or obese has serious long-term implications. If 2020 taught us anything, it's that we cannot put too high a price on our health. Extra weight triggers inflammation, which severely impacts immunity and how the body is able to deal with pathogens, like viruses. Ignored, it can also lead to the development of chronic conditions.

Factors like genetics have only a degree of influence on weight, so instead of saying, 'There's nothing I can do', we need to make better choices for ourselves. Weight loss is a science. Follow the methods properly and they will work without the need to radically change your life. Understanding the body is crucial, not only for losing weight, but keeping it off long-term.

# how to choose a weight-loss plan

Almost all of my patients want to lose weight and I have seen first-hand how much confusion there is around how to do it. The media is full of diets and theories, most of which would make a grown man cry and have no basis in medical research – but if a friend says they've had success with one, it's easy to think it might work for you too.

Most diets will succeed in achieving an initial drop in weight, no matter how silly they are, but this is really missing the point. Anyone can lose weight quickly, but if it's not done safely or with any understanding of nutrition and how the body functions, it will just as quickly go back on again. This kind of fluctuation is not good for the metabolism or for morale – I know this because I used to do it myself when I was working as a model. Quick-fix weight loss is unsustainable and can dangerously distort our relationship with food. We should enjoy what we eat, not be afraid of it.

# why all the body's systems are connected to weight loss

The human body is extraordinarily intelligent, making choices on your behalf every second of every day, but it can wander off track if not taken care of. As a clinician, I see so many people with other issues they don't realise are connected to their weight gain or inability to lose weight. If the body struggles with sleep, hormone imbalances, stress or nutritional deficiencies, it will never prioritise losing excess weight. That's why it's crucial when looking at healthy weight-loss plans to factor in the body as a whole, not just the areas of fat you'd like to get rid of.

I urge you to read all the chapters, because this knowledge will arm you with the tools to not only achieve your weight-loss goals but also maintain them and leave you feeling fantastic. All without giving up booze or chocolate. More on that later. Going forward, it's important not to be militant or hysterical about any kind of deviation. Having too many drinks or spending the afternoon lying on the sofa eating bread is not the end of the world. This is not Disney's Magic Kingdom. It's real life. Which can sometimes include hangovers.

*If you can't say goodbye to scales, use the digital kind that measure your body composition to give a more accurate reading on muscle–fat ratio and not just your weight.*

*Increasing beneficial fibre is easier than you think. Add a handful of greens to fruit smoothies and soups; use lettuce leaves instead of wraps and buns; or blitz up any type of non-starchy vegetable until it's tiny and add to literally anything – fried rice, pasta, shepherd's pie, fish pie, all the pies.*

# body composition – why it matters

The body is composed of fat, muscle, organs and bone mass. Muscle is heavier than fat because it is denser in volume, meaning that someone who is very muscular will be heavier than someone else of the same height and similar body shape but has less muscle and more fat.

Muscle is metabolically active tissue, which means it requires energy to function. Anything that requires muscle engagement – from standing, walking and talking to exercising – will involve the muscle cells burning glucose as energy. Fat tissue, on the other hand, is not metabolically active. Healthy weight loss, therefore, does involve losing excess fat – but it also means altering the body's composition to balance out the right muscle mass with appropriate levels of fat.

## the role of fat in the body

Everybody needs a certain amount of subcutaneous fat, which sits just under the skin. Very generally speaking, a healthy level should account for around 20–30 per cent of body weight, depending on age and gender. Fat's primary role is as a storage facility for energy. It's also essential for brain function, the central nervous system and to insulate and cushion the body.

## too much fat makes things go wrong

However, excess fat is unhealthy and can lead to illness. The more fat the body has, the more hormones it will secrete. Constantly signalling to the body that it is full starts to dull its impact, which drives up the desire to eat, resulting in the body storing more fat, and so on. Arrrghhh.

Fat also releases cytokines, the pro-inflammatory chemicals that contribute to systemic inflammation. In fact, research has revealed that obesity can actually be described as 'low-grade chronic inflammation' and this kind of inflammation is a known precursor to many chronic conditions. Then there's visceral fat, which is the kind stored around the midriff. Too much visceral fat puts stress on the abdomen's vital organs, with the potential to create more serious health conditions. The problems caused by being overweight extend way beyond the wardrobe.

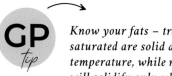

*Know your fats – trans and saturated are solid at room temperature, while monounsaturated will solidify only when chilled.*

*Scrub rather than peel vegetables and fruit. The skin is high in fibre, vitamins and minerals. Healthier and less work.*

# how does fat get formed?

When glucose (sugar) enters the bloodstream, the pancreas releases insulin, which carries it off to the cells in our muscle and liver. Insulin effectively opens the door to the cells for the glucose to enter and be converted into energy for immediate use. Any glucose that the body doesn't need to use straight away will be turned into glycogen and put away for later in the liver and muscle cells. There is a limit to how much both can store, so any excess will be transformed into triglycerides (a type of fat) and then stored in adipose tissue, which has no limit. And so there it sits.

Simple carbohydrates or foods that are high in sugar can eventually tire out the pancreas, as it keeps having to produce insulin, which gives the body the false impression that it has plenty of energy available for immediate use and does not need to burn anything reserved in its fat cells – in fact, it can go ahead and store more. This adds even further to weight gain.

# metabolism and basal metabolic rate

Metabolism refers to all the chemical processes in the body that are continually working to keep it alive, from cell repair to the conversion of food and drink into energy. The basal metabolic rate (BMR) refers to the daily number of calories the body uses when it is resting. Even in this state, it needs a constant supply of energy for all the jobs that are ongoing – circulation, breathing, thinking, adjusting hormone levels, growing and repairing cells. There are several factors that contribute to its calculation:

► **GENDER** – because men tend to have more muscle and less fat than women of their equivalent age and weight, they typically burn more calories.
► **AGE** – muscle usually begins to decrease with age, making way for more fat as calorie burning slows down.
► **BODY COMPOSITION AND SIZE** – people who are physically bigger or have more muscle burn more calories, even when they are relaxing.

The levels of energy the body requires for its resting state tend to stay relatively consistent and this is not something that can be easily changed. If a person's BMR is calculated as 1,000, it means their body will burn 1,000 calories each day just carrying out its basic functions to stay alive. There are other factors that will determine how many calories the body burns in a day:

► **THERMOGENESIS** – this refers to the amount of heat the body needs to generate to stay alive, which it produces by burning energy.
► **DIGESTION** – the body also produces heat during its digestive process, and this is believed to account for 3–10 per cent of calories used as energy.
► **PHYSICAL ACTIVITY** – deliberate movement, like walking, exercise or playing sport, will require the body to burn calories as fuel to create energy, and this will widely vary for each of us.

This means it's possible to eat more calories than the body's calculated BMR, as long as those calories are spent on physical activity and generating heat.

## what are calories?

Calories are units of energy provided in the form of heat by food and drink. The body, which is entirely energy-dependent, burns them and/or stores them as fuel. However, it's a little more complicated than just a numbers game. For example, 100 calories of broccoli and 100 calories of doughnut technically have the same energy value. Their nutritional value and effect on the body, on the other hand, is wildly different. Made of sugar and trans fats, doughnuts will lead to blood sugar spikes, crashes, cravings and eventually weight gain. Packed with fibre and nutrients, broccoli will keep blood sugar levels stabilised, helping the body to maintain a healthy weight. Refined and processed foods require almost no energy at all to be digested, which means most of their calorie content is absorbed into the body.

# what affects weight and metabolism?

## blood sugar levels

This is one of the easiest and quickest things to fix. I cannot stress enough how important balancing blood sugar levels is and what a difference it will make – to your weight, energy levels and overall health. The body uses the glucose it obtains from food to supply all its cells with the energy they require to function. When food is eaten, the body begins to digest and absorb its different particles into the bloodstream, including glucose, a simple sugar that is a component of carbohydrates. The speed at which glucose enters the blood will depend on several factors – what was eaten, when it was eaten and how it was eaten. These will all determine how blood sugar levels behave throughout the day – steady and balanced with mild fluctuations, or undulating wildly.

### BLOOD SUGAR BALANCE

There is a direct link between our blood sugar levels and how we feel. For example, are your energy levels steady and balanced or do you experience rollercoaster rushes of energy that are quickly followed by tiring dips? Blood sugar levels regulate everything – from mental health to cravings, appetite and sleep. When they are balanced, the body feels great. When they're not, it disrupts the equilibrium, causing chaos. Sounds miserable, because it is.

**WHAT** are you eating? Lacking in nutrients and stripped of their fibre, simple carbohydrates drive blood sugar levels up and excess unused glucose is stored as fat. Complex carbohydrates, which contain more fibre, are broken down and absorbed into the bloodstream more slowly.

**WHEN** are you eating? Eating regular meals plays a key role in blood sugar and the supply of energy, with healthy snacking in between preventing dips.

**HOW** are you eating? Macronutrients – protein, carbohydrates and fats – all require more complex processes to be broken down and eating them together slows and steadies the release of sugars into the bloodstream.

# unsustainable weight-loss plans

It's important to be realistic as any plan needs to fit around what is often a busy work and home life. Unrealistic programmes not only put people off more quickly but will also increase stress levels, which usually just results in more weight gained. Psychologically, deciding to go on a diet in the first place makes people much more aware of what they're eating, and the weight will come off. The problem is that so many of these plans are totally unsustainable and this is why approximately 80 per cent of diets fail. The odd fluctuation is absolutely normal and I always tell my patients to eat what they want at certain times of the year, like Christmas and holidays, because everyone needs to enjoy their lives. When general eating habits are better and healthier, losing a kilo or two again can be done without any dramatic changes.

# when the body negatively adapts

Crash diets or long-term restrictive calorie eating will cause the body to start adapting to the limited number of calories. This is why diets of this nature stop working: the metabolism will adjust by slowing down the rate at which it burns energy. Another problem is that they cause the body to lose weight too quickly and will include a loss of muscle mass, leading to a slower metabolism and lower metabolic rate. Crash diets train the body to work less efficiently at burning calories.

# stress, sleep and weight gain

The stress hormone cortisol has a significant effect on weight loss. Increased levels of cortisol can result in the body becoming resistant to insulin and this can lead to weight gain. If stress is chronic, it creates a vicious circle, increasing appetite and blood sugar levels. Cortisol also disrupts sleep, sending hormones spiralling, leading to cravings and weight gain.

# the intestinal microbiota

The digestive system is home to trillions of bacteria which play a crucial part in healthy digestion, cognitive and mental health, the immune system, appetite and energy levels. This flourishing micro-kingdom needs to be balanced to do its miraculous job properly but can easily be knocked off course by stress, poor sleep, the wrong kinds of food and medication. There is a strong link between an imbalanced microbiota and an inability to lose weight (see page 24).

# nature versus nurture

Our environment has a huge impact on our weight, from the diet we had as children to the family habits and attitudes we've picked up. While it's true that genetics plays a role in weight loss, this varies from person to person. Some research suggests that genes represent only about 25 per cent of a person's predisposition to gain weight. Genes can be influenced more than you think.

# So how do we do it?

## the balancing act

It's not possible to control absolutely everything you eat, unless you never want to go out and see your friends again. Everything is about balance. When so many of us are busy travelling, working and raising kids, coming up with a plan that is completely inflexible is only going to drive people mad and put them off. Keeping it simple is key. My goal is to educate you on the wide variety of delicious healthy food and correct eating habits that will leave you feeling better than ever.

## *the* GP principles

Get to know the importance of nutrients – how they work, where to find them and how best to eat them. The goal is that you'll end up energised, cheerful, hormonally balanced, sleeping like a dream and at a weight that's right for you.

### 1 PROTEIN

Amino acids are commonly referred to as the building blocks of proteins. It's their job to make new cells, repair damaged cells, oversee the production of hormones and neurotransmitters, support muscle growth and lean muscle mass and to ensure blood sugar and insulin levels are balanced. There are 20 amino acids that make proteins. The body can produce 11 of these itself, but we need to get the other 9 from our diet. To be considered 'complete', the protein we eat must contain all 9 essential amino acids.

### Animal proteins

Animal proteins are complete proteins. When possible, try to buy meat that has been raised on organic farms, is grass-fed, wild-caught or free-range. Buy well and less frequently:

▸ *Lean meat, poultry (turkey, chicken), fish (salmon, mackerel, white fish, tuna, sardines), shellfish (prawns, mussels, clams, oysters, crayfish, lobster), eggs and dairy products (milk, butter, cheese, yogurt).*

### Plant proteins

Some plant proteins are complete and particularly useful for vegetarians and vegans, especially fermented sources as they contain live bacteria that are highly beneficial for digestion. There are also many incredibly healthy sources that are incomplete, so combining them is essential:

▸ *Complete – quinoa, buckwheat, hemp and chia seeds, blue-green algae, (spirulina, chlorella and kelp), soy (edamame, tofu, tempeh, miso soup).*
▸ *Incomplete – whole grains (rye, spelt, wheat, oats), pulses (beans, chickpeas, lentils, peas).*

Easy ways to combine incomplete proteins:
▸ *Whole grains + beans (beans + brown rice, hummus + oatcakes, bean dip + crackers).*
▸ *Nuts or seeds + whole grains (nut butter on rye or pumpernickel bread).*
▸ *Beans or lentils + nuts or seeds (lentils/ chickpeas + pumpkin/sunflower seeds).*

*Protein portions for snacks just need to be a little smaller than meal portions. Let's say the palm and fist of a seven-year-old (as long as the seven-year-old you base this on is neither a giant nor a Lilliputian, but a child of distinctly average proportions).*

## How much protein should I eat?

I don't like being too specific about grams because everyone has different requirements. The most important thing to remember is that including protein in every meal or snack is essential. General guidance for a main meal:

▶ *Animal protein portions should be about the same size as the palm of your hand.*
▶ *Plant protein portions should be the same size as your fist.*

## a little note about dairy

I am not a huge fan of dairy, but I understand that some people can't imagine their lives without cheese. My advice is to go for organic when possible and choose different animal sources (less cow, more sheep and goat). Many people can develop dairy-related intolerances, as the proteins in cow's milk are larger and harder to digest, as opposed to sheep and goat's, which are smaller. Fermented dairy products are by far the best. This is because the fermentation process has effectively pre-digested the product, plus it contains beneficial bacteria:

▶ *Natural live yogurt, kefir, goat's and sheep cheeses.*
▶ *Dairy-free milks – nut (almond, cashew, hazelnut, coconut), oat, rice, soya, hemp; choose unsweetened milks with a high protein content, which will be listed on the label.*
▶ *Dairy-free alternatives are widely available, such as mozzarella and halloumi made from plants.*

## an even smaller note about nuts and seeds

Small but mighty, nuts and seeds are a powerful source of protein, as well as healthy fats, fibre, vitamins and minerals. They are such an easy snack option, either whole or in butter form:

▶ *Nuts – almonds, peanuts, Brazil, macadamias, hazelnuts, walnuts, cashews.*
▶ *Seeds – pumpkin, sunflower, chia, hemp, flax, sesame.*

*For a lighter kind of dip, swap sour cream as the base for natural yogurt or kefir, both of which come with plenty of beneficial bacteria that the intestine will love.*

*Nut butter can be eaten in so many ways. Try adding a spoonful to smoothies, cereal or, my personal favourite, porridge. It also makes a delicious dip for celery, pear or apple.*

*Starchy vegetables are higher in calories, so it's better to eat them during the day when you're more active and can use up the energy they provide, rather than in the evening, when, if you're anything like me, you're more likely to be lying on the sofa.*

## 2 CARBOHYDRATES

Made of starches, sugars and fibres, these are found in fruit, vegetables, grains, nuts, seeds and pulses. When the body digests carbohydrates, it breaks down their sugar and starch content into glucose, which is then absorbed into the bloodstream to be used and/or stored. They are the body's most crucial source of energy. However, some carbohydrates are more beneficial than others. The glycaemic index (GI) helps to determine the sugar and fibre content of carbohydrates, rating them from 0 to 100 according to how much they can elevate the blood sugar. The higher the number, the more quickly the carbohydrate is digested and absorbed, with the potential to spike blood sugar levels.

However, it's important to remember that the scale is an indication only, as higher GI foods will have their number reduced when eaten with proteins and fats. To take an example: white pasta is listed as a high-GI food, while wholegrain pasta is listed as lower because it contains more fibre. Eating either with other macronutrients – a protein like minced beef – will help reduce the GI rating for both of them. Wholegrain pasta still wins the low-GI prize. Don't get any ideas.

## Fibre – what's the big deal?

Essential for digestion, fibre is a type of carbohydrate found in plant-based foods. It helps to rid the body of toxins and anything that is redundant through excretion. There are two types of fibre and some foods contain both:

**Insoluble fibre** is found in the outer coating or skin of vegetables and whole grains, insoluble fibre helps to keep food moving in the intestines:

▸ *Fruit (often including skins and seeds) – (raspberries, pear, apples, strawberries, oranges, bananas, pomegranate), vegetables (peas, broccoli, cauliflower), nuts, seeds, lentils, beans, wholegrains (brown rice, buckwheat, quinoa, oats, barley).*

**Soluble fibre** slows the digestion process by attracting water like a magnet, helping to catch toxins, cholesterol and unwanted fats for excretion:

▸ *Oats, barley, nuts (almonds, cashews, hazelnuts, walnuts), seeds (flax, sunflower, pumpkin, chia), beans, lentils, fruit (blueberries, blackberries, raspberries, strawberries, pears, kiwis, plums, figs, apricots), vegetables (spinach, avocado, sweet potato, broccoli, carrots).*

*White rice is brown rice that has had its coat robbed and then been bleached, taking all the fibre and most of its nutritional value with it. Brown rice – including my favourite, pre-cooked type – is a quick and easy alternative and especially good with takeaways.*

*For those avoiding gluten, don't forget there are naturally gluten-free grains, such as buckwheat, brown rice, millet and quinoa. Stay away from the highly processed, bleached products which scream 'NO FIBRE'.*

## Grains

Grains are seeds that come from two sources – cereal plants (oats, rice, wheat) and pseudo cereal plants (buckwheat, quinoa, amaranth). When eaten in their whole form (wholegrains), they are very healthy, as they tend to be high in nutrients like fibre, magnesium, B vitamins, iron, phosphorus, manganese and selenium. Like a bad out-of-town cousin who taught you how to smoke, refined grains are a less wholesome story. Stripped of fibre and nutrients, they are referred to as 'empty calories' and don't have much to offer. Sad face.

- *Wholegrains include oats, barley, millet, quinoa, brown rice, whole wheat, bulgur.*
- *Refined grains include white-flour products (white bread, croissants, baguette), white rice, white pasta, pastries.*

## a note on vegetables

Some of my clients are surprised that all vegetables are carbohydrates. What makes them especially beneficial is that they tend to be high in fibre and low in sugar, and have a low GI, as well as being rich in vitamins and minerals. There are two types of vegetable – starchy, which is higher in calories, and non-starchy. To compare in a very general sense, a cooked portion of starchy corn is about 80 calories, while the same portion size of non-starchy cauliflower would contain around 25 calories. Don't hate me, corn fan club.

- *Starchy vegetables – potatoes, corn, parsnips, beans, peas, butternut squash, chickpeas, lentils.*
- *Non-starchy vegetables – broccoli, kale, cauliflower, cabbage, asparagus, beansprouts, chard, bok choy, Brussels sprouts, artichokes, aubergine, cucumber, spinach, courgette.*

## another note on fruit

Fruit and fruit juices. Are they healthy? Are they too sugary? The general rule is to use common sense. The sweeter the fruit, the more sugar it contains. Similarly, the more fruit needs to be chewed is a good sign, as it means the fibre content is higher. Hurray.

- *High fibre – apples, passion fruit, pear, kiwi, blueberries, raspberries, pineapple.*
- *Low fibre – cantaloupe, watermelon, nectarine, papaya, peaches.*

All fruit contains many fantastically healthy phytonutrients, antioxidants, vitamins, minerals and soluble fibre. Most have a very high water content (sometimes up to 95 per cent), making them a source of hydration. Also good. The ones that appear higher on the GI index should be considered more of a treat than their lower-GI pals, but in general, fresh, raw fruit is an amazing source of nutrients that should be eaten regularly.

*Eating fruit on an empty stomach will cause blood sugar spikes, so always have it with or after food, or as a snack with a protein source like nuts, seeds or live yogurt. And with drinks, blend rather than juice to keep the pulp and fibre.*

*White fluffy bread and pastries may try to charm you with their crusty, warm deliciousness, but that's just part of their evil plan to seduce you and then leave you with nothing. Look out for seeds and nuts in darker bread, because the denser and chewier it is, the better.*

## a really tiny note on bread

Bread is not what it used to be. Due to high demand, its mass production has led to the creation of something that has almost entirely lost connection to its natural source. The best bread resembles what people were making before chemicals and factories got involved. Dark rye or pumpernickel is like eating nutrient-rich seeds and grains stuck together and is a far superior alternative.

## 3 FATS

Fats probably wish they'd been born with a more appealing name, as they are actually an essential part of a healthy diet. Fat is needed for the growth of all the body's cells, forming a large percentage of cell membranes, providing energy, protecting the organs and keeping the body warm. Without it, the body cannot absorb fat-soluble vitamins like A, D and E. Diets that are low in fat do not fill the body up. This can lead to cravings and overeating, as the body never feels satisfied. Fat-free foods are also highly misleading as the removed fat is often replaced with refined sugar. This can influence weight gain, with the body having to convert all the excess sugar into triglycerides, which are stored in fat cells. However, it's important to note that while some fats are critical for the body to function properly, there are some that are not. These different types range from scoundrel to hero, with a few complex characters in between.

## Worst: trans fatty acids

Trans fats can be found in some meat and dairy, but these are natural and not worth getting too worried about. The real villains are the artificial kind. Found predominantly in hydrogenated vegetable oils, they are used a lot in manufactured foods, like cakes, biscuits and fast foods, to prolong shelf life and maintain flavour. They can increase the risk of heart disease and strokes by raising levels of LDL (bad cholesterol), which builds up in the arteries, making them narrower and harder, and reducing HDL (good cholesterol), which is important for escorting excess cholesterol back to the liver. Trans fatty acids can lead to weight gain and the subsequent risk factors for many chronic conditions like diabetes and cancer:

▸ *Fried food (French fries, doughnuts), margarine, shop-bought baked goods (biscuits, cakes, pastries), frozen pizza, processed snacks (microwave popcorn).*

*'Partially hydrogenated' indicates that the oils in the ingredients have been solidified into trans fats, like the kind found in margarine. Put the margarine down and leave. As for doughnuts – what can I say? Don't eat doughnuts.*

*Use extra virgin, walnut and flax oils for dressings. When buying, keep an eye out for 'cold pressed', 'unrefined' and 'expeller pressed' on the label, as this indicates a higher quality.*

*Polyunsaturated fats deteriorate rapidly in light and warmth, so keep omega-3 supplements (the liquid form, as this doesn't apply to the capsules), flax and hemp oil in the fridge.*

*I like using rapeseed, coconut oil or ghee for high-heat cooking. Coconut oil is also fantastic for baking, as it works really well in sweet foods. Not that you're going to be eating many of those from now on, LOL.*

## Mixed feelings: saturated fats

Saturated fats get a bad press, but they are also important to many processes in the body, as long as they are eaten in moderation. These include supporting healthy bones, improving the immune system, balancing digestive microflora and assisting the liver with processing alcohol and other toxins:

▸ *Fatty cuts of meat (lamb, pork, beef, dark poultry meat and skin), high-fat dairy (whole milk, butter, cheese, ice cream), lard and tropical oils (coconut, palm).*

## The middlemen: monounsaturated fats

Monounsaturated fats can help with weight loss, improve insulin sensitivity and support immunity, all of which also reduce the risk of heart disease. In fact, research suggests that eating just half a tablespoon of olive oil a day can lower the risk of cardiovascular disease by around 15 per cent:

▸ *Olive oil, avocados, nuts (almonds, cashews, peanuts, pistachios), seeds (pumpkin, sunflower), eggs.*

## Obsessed: polyunsaturated fatty acids

Polyunsaturated fats are classified as essential fatty acids, the only kind of fats the body is unable to produce itself. This is why it's critical to include plenty in the diet, as this is the only way the body can obtain them. Imagine this sentence is underlined in red pen, ten feet tall and on fire. Extremely important. Today's diets include a lot more omega-6 fatty acids than they used to, but these acids are known to increase inflammation – and while we need inflammation to protect the body when injured, too much of it might lead to imbalances.

Conversely, omega-3 fatty acids contain highly effective anti-inflammatory properties. Keeping a balanced ratio between these fatty acids is the key to benefiting from their capabilities:

▸ *Omega-3: fish (mackerel, herring, salmon, trout, sardines, tuna), shellfish (prawns, mussels, clams, crayfish, oysters), nuts (walnuts, almonds, macadamia, hazelnuts, pecans), seeds (pumpkin, sunflower, hemp, chia, flax).*
▸ *Omega-6: vegetable oils (safflower, sunflower, walnut, soybean).*

*Always go for high-quality fish oil supplements, as cheaper versions like cod liver oil can contain impurities and toxins.*

*For vegans and non-fish eaters, try omega-3 supplements made from nutrient-packed algae.*

## 4 PHYTONUTRIENTS

In addition to their extremely high micronutrient levels (vitamins and minerals), plants also contain phytonutrients, the compounds found in all their edible elements, particularly the skin or peel. They are what give plants their smell, colour and taste – rocket its bitterness, beetroot its redness and chillies their heat. Research continues to reveal just how beneficial phytochemicals are.

Flavonoids in lemons and pears may have anti-inflammatory properties, and anthocyanins in berries and red wine are believed to lower blood pressure. Catechins in green tea can reduce the risk of cancer, and sulphides in onions, shallots, garlic and leeks contain antibacterial and antifungal properties and may help boost immunity. Eating a rainbow of different-coloured plants is the best way to get the full range of their benefits.

## Cooked, raw or frozen?

There can be a certain amount of confusion around which foods are best to eat raw or cooked. The general rule is eat seasonally and use a combination – more raw foods during the warmer months and cooked foods when it's colder. Organic is always better, when possible. Scrub the skin, rather than peeling, as it contains high levels of antioxidants that will otherwise be lost.

While cooking methods like boiling will damage the nutritional content of the food, steaming can actually increase vital nutrients, antioxidants and vitamins and make them more digestible. Use very little water and steam until tender (but not soft) and the colour has been retained. Some plant foods like nuts and seeds will benefit from being soaked overnight. This activates the nutrient content and makes them easier to digest.

It's always a good idea to have frozen fruit and vegetables to hand (my freezer is rammed with them), as it means you never have an excuse for leaving them out. The higher the quality when they were frozen, the better they will keep their nutritional content.

You need to know about one of my obsessions. Sprouted grains or seeds, such as mung beans, broccoli, kale and alfalfa, are highly potent sources of activated goodness. Low in calories and incredibly rich in fibre, enzymes, protein, phytonutrients and micronutrients, they are like tiny nutrient explosions.

*Don't think smoothies have to just be fruit – they actually work brilliantly with many types of vegetables. Try adding a handful of something green and/or leafy, as whizzing up a rainbow blend of plant sources is an easy way to ensure a hearty phytochemical fix.*

*Add sprouted grains or seeds to salads, soups, sandwiches, stir-fries (also applicable to foods that don't start with 's').*

*Always have a bag of mixed frozen berries in the freezer – they're so handy for smoothies and home-made ice cream.*

## Herbs and spices

Include as many herbs and spices as you like when cooking – the more, the merrier – as they add a huge variety of flavours and have been used across the centuries for their medicinal properties and myriad health benefits, which we're continuing to learn about:

- *Parsley* – bright and peppery, parsley aids blood clotting, helps keep bones healthy, supports immunity and can reduce the risk of heart disease.
- *Ginger* – fiery and cleansing, it has a well-documented calming effect on irritated stomachs and nausea. It can protect cells against oxidation and is anti-inflammatory.
- *Peppermint* – fresh and cool, the oil in the leaves has been shown to soothe abdominal cramps, reduce bloating and support digestive health.

- *Garlic* – while it's technically a vegetable, the chemical compound allicin, its active ingredient, is known to be antimicrobial and can help fight off bacteria and viruses as well as balance intestinal flora.
- *Cinnamon* – earthy and warm, it is sweet, but not calorific and can defend against free radicals and pathogenic bacteria.
- *Turmeric* – rich in the powerful free-radical-slaying curcumin, this woody yellow spice boosts the body's own antioxidant enzymes and is an important natural anti-inflammatory. It has been shown to lower the risk of heart disease and cancer, as well as improve brain and cognitive function.
- *Chillies* – their hot active ingredient capsaicin is known to boost metabolism.
- *Cardamom* – citrusy and aromatic, it is rich in magnesium and zinc and has been shown to help ease excessive inflammation.

*Keep herbs fresh for longer by freezing them in ziplock sachets or ice cube trays inside a bag to prevent freezer burn.*

*Two teaspoons of turmeric mixed in a jar of honey is divine. Spread a thin layer on top of nut-buttered grainy toast.*

## The importance of hydration

On average, humans are composed of over 50 per cent water. The body needs water for all kinds of essential systems and processes, like transporting nutrients, oxygen and glucose to cells, supporting skin, joint, eye and digestive health, and flushing toxins and waste out through the kidneys.

We also need water for our inner thermostat, especially during hot weather or physical activity like exercise. Fluids the body loses through sweat produced to regulate our temperature will need to be replaced, as low fluid levels can lead to headaches, exhaustion, lack of focus, light-headedness and constipation. Keeping fluid levels topped up is also important for weight loss, as dehydration can sometimes feel like hunger. Adults should drink between 1.5–2.5 litres (8–12 cups) of water a day. This will vary, though, depending on levels of physical activity and how hot the weather is, so regularly drinking fluids and not ignoring feelings of thirst is important.

*To make water more exciting, try flavouring it with citruses, ginger, cucumber or mint. I also love kombucha and apple cider vinegar drinks, which come in lots of delicious different flavours.*

## The two faces of caffeine

While coffee is rich in powerful antioxidants, caffeine can sometimes be regarded as rather a shady character. Research suggests that coffee can lower the risk of developing some chronic illnesses, in addition to supporting several brain functions – mood, energy levels, memory and focus. It can also boost the body's metabolic rate, stimulate the nervous system and trigger fat cells to release stored fatty acids from adipose tissue.

HANG ON, THOUGH. Come closer, because this is a story of two halves. Caffeine can also be addictive, especially if more than four caffeinated cups are drunk in a day. Reducing it can be hard, with withdrawal symptoms including headaches, tiredness, muscle pain and cravings. Caffeine also triggers the release of the stress hormones, cortisol and adrenaline. These stimulate the liver to flood the bloodstream with glucose in the same way it would if you were confronted with a pack of wolves. The body behaves as if it is in emergency mode, unable to tell the difference between a genuine threat and a double espresso, resulting in spiked blood sugar levels.

▶ *Coffee is not something I tell people to cut out. What I do suggest is managing intake and always combining it with a protein-rich snack or meal.*
▶ *Caffeine behaves differently from person to person, so having an awareness of its effects will help us benefit from its good qualities and minimise its negative effects.*

**GP**
*Tip*

*White and green tea are a great alternative to coffee as they contain less caffeine, so you don't have to go cold turkey. They are also packed with more antioxidants than you can shake a stick at.*

# The GP principles recapped

▶ Eat a portion of protein with every meal, including snacks.

▶ Choose carbohydrates that are high in fibre with a lower GI.

▶ Include a variety of healthy fats, with a focus on essential fatty acids.

▶ Keep fluid levels topped up regularly throughout the day.

▶ Try to avoid drinking caffeine on an empty stomach.

▶ Increase the diversity of phytonutrients with a rainbow diet.

▶ Maintain blood sugar balance by eating when peckish, not starving.

▶ Don't skip meals and include balanced snacks.

# intermittent fasting

So *drumroll* here we go. The two intermittent fasting (IF) plans to help you meet your weight-loss goals and feel fantastic. AT LAST. In all my years practising as a nutritionist, these have been, without question, the most effective ways of delivering quick, sustainable results that fit simply into anyone's lifestyle.

IF has decades of scientific research behind it to prove that it works and I have seen first-hand the profound changes it makes, both physically and mentally. This method is easy, sustainable and realistic for every lifestyle. Aside from being extremely effective for weight loss, it has numerous other health benefits – for example, better blood sugar control, greater energy levels, improved sleep, a reduction in the risk of chronic and age-related diseases and an increase in lifespan.

Use of the word 'fast' makes people think they can't eat at all, but these IF plans work differently. The first plan involves introducing a significant calorie restriction for three days a week, while the other has a daily fasting window of 16 hours (including overnight, which means sleeping through a large part of it). The good news is, nobody is going to starve until they keel over and fade away. You will be eating, don't worry.

## why intermittent fasting?

IF helps the body lose weight without impacting the basal metabolic rate or reducing muscle mass. This means these fasting plans won't cause metabolic adaptation. During fasting, the body consumes less energy. With insulin's job slowed down, its levels drop and the body turns to its glycogen stores in the liver for energy, followed by fat stores in adipose tissue. This is how the weight starts to come off.

Alternating between fasting and healthy eating means the body does not stay in this energy deficit for long and our metabolism remains stable. IF improves insulin sensitivity, which means the body is more efficient at balancing blood sugar levels, making it very beneficial for people who are at risk of diabetes or cardiovascular disease. IF and weight loss have also been shown to decrease levels of inflammation, while sharpening memory, mood and cognitive function.

This one is my favourite. IF stimulates a process known as autophagy ('auto' meaning self and 'phagy' meaning self-devouring). Before you start having nightmares that your body is going to start eating itself, this refers to something really quite extraordinary. Autophagy is an evolutionary form of self-preservation. The body goes into reset mode, clearing out redundant and damaged cells in order to repair and regenerate new cells, which is particularly beneficial for ageing. The body emerges as a greater expression of itself.

# why not restrict calories?

The logical question would be, 'Why don't I just eat less all the time?' The downside of continuous calorie-restriction diets is that the body will get used to a decreased calorie intake and become reluctant to turn to its long-term energy stores in adipose tissue. Another downside is that the body can turn to the muscle tissue itself as a source of energy, breaking it down and therefore negatively impacting body composition.

## a little note on intermittent fasting and blood sugar levels

Blood sugar balance is crucial to maintaining good health. However, within the context of these weight-loss programmes, it is essential that blood sugar levels drop, so that the body can then turn to stored fat reserves, breaking them down as a source of energy. This is all part of a perfectly normal biochemical process, but it's important to note that it is only recommended as part of IF specifically.

## Superhero nutrients

**Along with a good-quality multi-nutrient (see page 204) as a baseline for all daily requirements, consider some of these:**

- **Soluble fibre (Glucomannan and psyllium husk)** – attracts water and forms a gel-like substance in the stomach. It naturally helps you to feel fuller for longer, balances blood sugar levels and feeds healthy bacteria in the intestine.

- **Probiotics** – keeps the vital intestinal microbiota balanced, which amongst many other benefits assists with healthy weight loss and appetite control.

- **Chromium** – a mineral that increases the efficiency of insulin as it transports glucose to the cells for energy, helping to stabilise blood sugar levels and reduce cravings.

- **B vitamins** – essential for balancing energy levels. They support healthy metabolism to ensure the body uses the glucose from our food as energy, rather than storing it as triglycerides in adipose tissue.

- **Green tea extract** – rich in antioxidants and phytochemicals, this has not only been shown to reduce inflammation and support the immune system, it can assist with the breakdown and release of stored fat in adipose tissue during the weight-loss process.

# introducing the GP 4:3 and GP 16:8

Both IF plans will provide the same health benefits. The point of having two plans is to allow you to choose which one suits you, your lifestyle and your weight-loss goals the best. These plans are extremely effective. Changes can start to appear after a few days, but two weeks is the minimum for the body to begin to make real adjustments. Each person's current weight, associated goals, the state of their health and how their body responds, will vary, as we are not all identikit robots from the same factory, who function in exactly the same way. The beauty of both these plans is that they are healthy, safe and easy to keep going with until all targets are reached.

## the 4:3 plan

- ▶ A more restricted programme for significant targeted weight loss.

- ▶ Easier to follow for people who plan their week in advance.

- ▶ **FASTING DAYS:** 500 calories for women / 600 for men on 3 non-consecutive days over the course of a week.

- ▶ **MINDFUL DAYS:** follow the GP principles for healthy eating, trying to reduce the amount eaten a little (by about 20%).

- ▶ **MAGIC DAY:** one day a week where no restrictions apply and you can eat what you like.

People generally find 4:3 easier than they thought it would be, with some noticing that anything from energy levels to sleep can improve quickly. It's also true that there are days that might feel tougher, because making changes requires self-control, which some will find easier than others. Experiencing dips and the occasional energy and mood wobbles are also completely normal, as the body goes through a process of reorganising itself, but don't be discouraged – this is meant to happen. Almost everyone experiences a version of it.

The tables and delicious nutrient-rich recipes in chapter 11 have all been designed to make the plan clear and simple to follow. In all the years I have been putting clients on 4:3, it has worked – without exception. Every one of them has come to the end feeling ten times better. I know you will too.

# your two-week 4:3 schedule

It's important to note that day 14 is the only exception to the schedule. As the last day of the plan, it should be a mindful day. There is only one magic day in the two weeks.

| DAY 1 | Monday | Fasting day | 500 (f) 600 (m) |
|---|---|---|---|
| DAY 2 | Tuesday | Mindful day | GP principles* |
| DAY 3 | Wednesday | Fasting day | 500 (f) 600 (m) |
| DAY 4 | Thursday | Mindful day | GP principles* |
| DAY 5 | Friday | Fasting day | 500 (f) 600 (m) |
| DAY 6 | Saturday | Mindful day | GP principles* |
| DAY 7 | Sunday | MAGIC DAY!!! | No restrictions |
| DAY 8 | Monday | Fasting day | 500 (f) 600 (m) |
| DAY 9 | Tuesday | Mindful day | GP principles* |
| DAY 10 | Wednesday | Fasting day | 500 (f) 600 (m) |
| DAY 11 | Thursday | Mindful day | GP principles* |
| DAY 12 | Friday | Fasting day | 500 (f) 600 (m) |
| DAY 13 | Saturday | Mindful day | GP principles* |
| DAY 14 | Sunday | Mindful day | GP principles* |

*= intake reduced by 20%*

# fasting day advice

## Plan your meals
Divide your calorie allowance to suit both your schedule and preferences. Try to space them out between two or three small meals or one meal and a couple of snacks. Alternatively, some people prefer to save all their calories for one larger evening meal.

## Stay hydrated
Thirst can often be confused with hunger, so it's very important to stay hydrated on fasting days. Drink at least two litres of water or non-caffeinated liquids a day.

## Meal composition
Follow the GP principles with smaller portions and stay within the calorie limit (see pages 130–75 for fasting day recipe ideas):
- *Include a portion of protein with every meal.*
- *Avoid simple carbohydrates. Choose high-fibre carbohydrates, especially non-starchy vegetables, as they're low in calories and will keep you fuller for longer.*
- *Avoid high-fat foods, like oil, butter, cheese and avocado, as they are nutrient-dense and will bring you up to your calorie allowance without making you feel full.*

# mindful day advice

Follow the GP principles for each meal, making portions around 20 per cent smaller than normal (see page 25). Alternatively, you could reduce your overall calorie intake by 20% for the day, e.g. a normal-size breakfast and lunch, a snack and then finishing with a very light dinner. An example of a nicely balanced meal:
- *½ non-starchy vegetables (broccoli, kale, spinach).*
- *¼ whole grains (brown rice, quinoa, rye) or starchy vegetables (potatoes, corn, peas).*
- *¼ protein (fish, poultry, tofu).*

## FREQUENTLY ASKED QUESTIONS

**Q: Do I need to start this plan on a Monday?**
Starting on a Monday is recommended, because this means the magic day can be at the weekend. It's totally your choice, though.

**Q: Can I switch fasting and mindful days?**
Absolutely – the main point is that you have to fast for three non-consecutive days in a week.

**Q: Can I have two mindful days in a row?**
Yes – Monday, Wednesday, Friday tends to be easier as the fasting days, but Monday, Wednesday and Saturday is an alternative, which will leave two mindful days on Thursday and Friday.

**Q: What is a magic day?**
A magic day is one day off within the two-week plan, here you can relax and forget about following any restrictions with what you eat.

**Q: Does my magic day have to be a Sunday?**
No. You can swap any one of the mindful days with the magic day, but just remember that you only get one magic day in the two-week plan.

**Q: What if I am finding it tough and eat more on a fasting day?**
If you've eaten significantly more calories on a fasting day, count that as a mindful day and resume fasting the next day.

**Q: What about exercise?**
It's technically fine to exercise on a fasting day, but it really comes down to how you feel, with gentler forms of exercise a preferable option.

**Q: What about alcohol?**
Alcohol is not recommended for fasting days, as it will impact your restricted-calorie intake for the day. When it comes to mindful days, the decision is ultimately personal – although the calories remain high.

# *the* 16:8 plan

▸ A less-restricted programme for milder weight loss and weight-loss maintenance.

▸ Easier to follow for people who are less inclined to plan and have busy, unpredictable schedules.

▸ 16 hours of fasting (including overnight).

▸ 8 non-fasting hours following the GP principles.

▸ Healthy eating as opposed to calorie counting.

This plan is incredibly straightforward and involves no planning ahead like the 4:3. The 16-hour fasting window is partially overnight, which means you'll sleep through a large part of it. Then it's just a question of following the GP principles for eating healthy, balanced meals over the remaining 8 hours of the day.

It is designed for those who are less focused on targeted, significant weight loss. You will lose weight if you need to (bodies are so clever), but it's a slower, gentler approach. It tends to work better for those who only want to lose a few pounds or maintain a healthy weight – although it also acts as an incredible reset for the body, leaving it feeling reinvigorated and super-charged.

## FREQUENTLY ASKED QUESTIONS

**Q: What should I eat during my 8-hour window?**
Follow the GP principles for healthy eating (see page 22). For an example of a nicely balanced meal (see page 27).

**Q: Do I have to stick to the same times?**
No – it's completely up to you to decide when to start the eating window each day.

**Q: When is the best time to exercise?**
Some people are fine exercising during periods of fasting, but I would suggest you only do any high-intensity training during your 8-hour eating window. Others find they prefer gentler forms of exercise. Listen to your body.

**Q: Can I still have caffeine?**
▸ Eating window – *follow the GP principles and always have your caffeinated drink with or after a balanced meal or snack.*
▸ Fasting window – *it's preferable to avoid caffeine and try herbal teas, but if that is unbearable, try not to have more than one caffeinated drink with no milk or sugar.*

**Q: What about alcohol?**
Alcohol is high in calories, so it would be better to cut back. If you do have a drink, make sure it's during your 8-hour eating window.

# planning your 8-hour eating window

**EARLY BIRDS:** If you prefer not to miss breakfast, eat in the morning and finish late afternoon. I would recommend going to bed early to avoid feeling hungry in the evening.

| FASTING | 8-hour eating window 10am–6pm | FASTING |
|---|---|---|
| WAKE UP<br><br>MORNING PART OF YOUR 16-HOUR FAST | 10am: first meal<br><br>1pm: snack/small meal<br><br>5pm: last meal | EVENING PART OF YOUR 16-HOUR FAST<br><br>SLEEPING |

**MIDDLE-OF-THE-DAY BIRDS:** If you're happy to skip breakfast and prefer to have lunch and dinner at a more normal time, start at midday.

| FASTING | 8-hour eating window 12pm–8pm | FASTING |
|---|---|---|
| WAKE UP<br><br>MORNING PART OF YOUR 16-HOUR FAST | 12pm: first meal<br><br>3.30pm: snack/small meal<br><br>7pm: last meal | EVENING PART OF YOUR 16-HOUR FAST<br><br>SLEEPING |

**NIGHT OWLS:** Start with a slightly later lunch and extend into the evening. This is the best option for those who have evening engagements.

| FASTING | 8-hour eating window 2pm–10pm | FASTING |
|---|---|---|
| WAKE UP<br><br>MORNING PART OF YOUR 16-HOUR FAST | 2pm: first meal<br><br>5pm: snack/small meal<br><br>9pm: last meal | EVENING PART OF YOUR 16-HOUR FAST<br><br>SLEEPING |

# 2/

# the power
*of* immunity

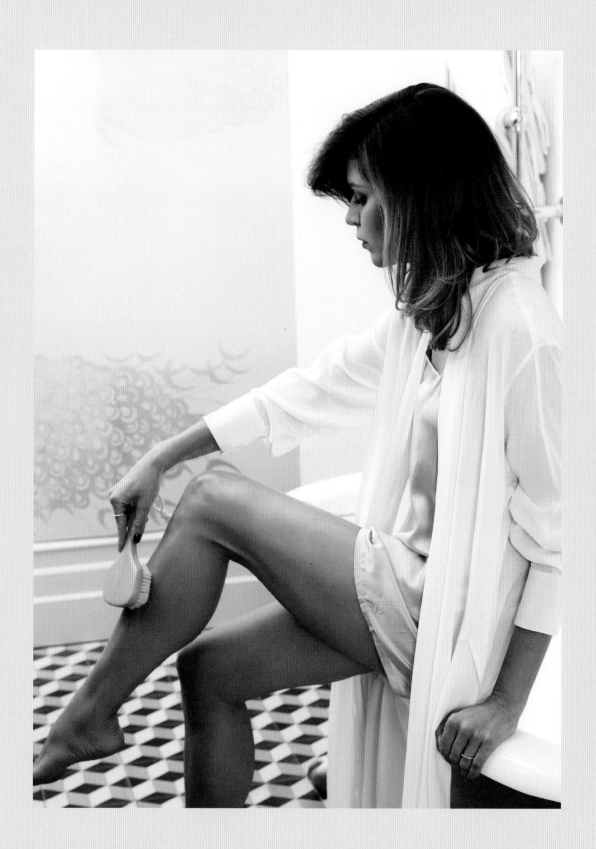

*do you* ...

- ☐ get colds more frequently than others?
- ☐ take a while to get better after an illness?
- ☐ regularly take antibiotics?
- ☐ suffer from allergies including hay fever?
- ☐ find you are prone to conditions like eczema or psoriasis?

# what is the immune system?

It is not an understatement to say that the human body houses the most sophisticated form of organised protection in the world. The body's immunity is a highly intelligent system that is able to recognise literally millions of pathogens (glam word for germs), distinguishing them from the body's own healthy cells and destroying each one in a targeted response.

An intricate network of organs, cells and chemicals, the immune system is in constant communication with itself. It responds quickly to any identified threat from a pathogen by mobilising the immune cells or chemicals that are nearest to the problem, dispatching them as swiftly as possible to deal with the situation.

During this process, the reaction of the immune system may result in us feeling more unwell while it gets to work. The symptoms of a cold or fever are not just caused by the invading virus. Sweating helps eliminate toxins and swelling is a sign of increased blood flow, both of which are better environments for the immune cells to initiate the attack. Sometimes it has to be cruel to be kind.

Once the enemy has been vanquished, the immune system will then remember its encounter with this particular pathogen, meaning that should it have the audacity to show up again, it will be recognised and destroyed with an even more ruthless efficiency.

# the villains and heroes

The immune system is a complicated, interconnected structure comprised of nodes, ducts, glands, tonsils and the spleen. It distributes immune cells throughout the body via the blood and lymphatic system, working as one unit to identify and deal with pathogens.

Lymphatic fluid contains pathogen-destroying white blood cells. These white blood cells are stored in lymph nodes, which work like checkpoints throughout the lymphatic system. Suspicious pathogens such as viruses and bacteria will be stopped at the lymph nodes, which is why swollen glands are often a symptom of the body fighting infection. It is a sign that high numbers of white blood cells are congregating in order to launch a counterattack.

## the villains – and how we find them

Pathogens, or germs, come in many forms, most commonly bacteria, viruses and fungi. Antigens form part of their structure, existing on the surface, but are also found on non-living foreign bodies, like toxins and chemicals. Antigens are like a stamp on these invaders, enabling their identification as harmful.

### VIRUSES
Viruses, like Covid-19, mumps, measles and rubella, are forms of genetic code which are protected by a protein coating. They are unable to reproduce on their own, so once they get into the body, they need to find a host cell to attach to; then they multiply. They are then released from the host cell, which will be left damaged or dead, to continue on their rampage to infect more cells. Even after the body appears to have recovered, some viruses can remain dormant, only to re-emerge and multiply again.

### BACTERIA
Bacteria are single-cell microorganisms of different shapes and features that can live in just about any environment on or in the body. Not all bacteria are bad (like our intestinal microbiota), but others can cause infections with varying degrees of seriousness. Bacterial infections include urinary tract infections (UTIs), strep throat, bacterial pneumonia (it can also be viral), salmonella, listeria and E. coli.

### FUNGI
There are millions of different types of fungus in the environment, but many are harmless. Fungi are protected by a thick cell wall, which makes them hard to kill. Candida is an increasingly common fungal infection; it's linked to higher sugar levels in the diet, amongst other things.

*Fevers are the body's way of helping to flush out pathogens and stimulate the immune response. If possible, let nature run its course with mild fevers in adults. Seek medical help if the fever increases or doesn't improve.*

*Boost the immune system during the colder months with a vitamin D supplement, minimum 10mcg (400IU) per day. If you feel you need more due to factors like less sun exposure, do a simple blood test with a GP (not me, a doctor).*

# two immune systems are better than one

## INNATE IMMUNE RESPONSE

The body is born with an innate immunity – an in-built surveillance system that works as the general defence against most day-to-day pathogens through physical and chemical barriers (coughing, tears, skin, mucus and stomach acid). It doesn't develop a memory for past invaders, but does work very quickly to deal with threats.

## ACQUIRED IMMUNE RESPONSE

This is not something the body is born with, but something it learns. When a pathogen enters the body and cannot be dealt with by the innate immune response, the expert cells will step in and launch an entirely bespoke attack designed to deal with the unique threat. While it's initially slower to respond, the acquired immune response's great gift is its memory. It will memorise its attack as part of its ability to learn, adapt and retain information. When the same adversary returns, the acquired immune response is immediately able to recognise it, remember how it was initially dealt with and destroy it much more quickly and efficiently than it did the first time. This is the principle on which vaccinations work, when a micro-dose of a dead or weakened pathogen is introduced into the body in order to create cell memory in the immune system, so that any future invasions are swiftly crushed.

## but wait... are we all too clean?

Studies suggest that having smaller families, less contact with animals, and houses that are cleaned to the point of sterilisation, has become detrimental to our health as our immune systems cannot develop properly. Immune systems are strengthened through their own learning process, especially in childhood. So, if you see your child licking the dog, don't pull up a chair and cheer them on, but don't panic either. Their immunity might actually benefit.

## the heroes and what they do

The immune response consists of an army of highly sophisticated white blood cells that love nothing more than to bring down an attempted invasion. Made in the bone marrow, they are stored in blood and lymph tissue and survive for 1–3 days. In spite of the fact that the bone marrow is constantly producing them, their numbers are very low. Their impact, however, is enormous as immune cells have unique roles. They include phagocytes, the everyday cleaners, which go around like Pac-Men, munching up commonplace pathogens. However, more serious threats, like viruses or infections, activate a spectacular specialised response, where they are memorised and disabled by B cells and destroyed by T cells and Natural Killer cells. This learned response means the immune system will know how to deal with any repeat invasion by the same troublemakers.

*To stimulate the lymph's white blood cell circulation, dry-brush the skin with a natural bristle brush. Use long strokes towards the heart, going over each area two or three times to fire up your inner bodyguards.*

# immunity & intestinal microflora

The immune system and intestinal tract are tightly interlinked and their relationship is incredibly important. The intestine houses around 70 per cent of the body's immune system in its gut-associated lymphoid tissue, or GALT for short. The immune system evolves to recognise the trillions of healthy bacteria that live in the intestine as safe and leave them unharmed. In turn these healthy bacteria influence the development of the immune system.

# antioxidants & free radicals

This is a story of theft and self-sacrifice. Free radicals are unstable molecules that are natural by-products of biochemical reactions in the body. They are also used by the immune system to help fight pathogens. We are constantly generating free radicals in response to stimulants – for example, substances in the food we eat, UV rays, pollution and tobacco smoke.

What makes free radicals problematic is that they contain only one electron, so they are unstable. Electrons like being in pairs, so free radicals travel around the body trying to steal electrons from other cells to make up a pair, leaving these mugged cells damaged. It is normal for the body to produce free radicals, as long as their numbers are balanced. If levels become too high, they can be harmful and lead to health problems. This is where antioxidants come in. Antioxidants are compounds that selflessly hand over their own electrons to free radicals, which neutralises them and stops them robbing other cells. True altruists.

# inflammation

Acute inflammation is a vital part of the immune response to injury or tissue damage. The immune system releases inflammatory mediators, including histamine and bradykinin, which stimulate blood vessels to dilate, increasing blood flow to damaged tissue so that more immune cells can be rushed on-site to start the healing process. This increased blood and fluid to the area is usually accompanied by redness and swelling. Similarly, a blocked or stuffy nose is the result of mucous membranes in the nasal passages becoming inflamed and generating more fluid. This excess fluid can assist in flushing viruses, bacteria and allergens out of the body.

## ▶ CHRONIC INFLAMMATION

Chronic inflammation is a different story altogether and is the result of an inflammatory response being unable to recover from whatever is causing the problem. This could be anything from viruses, bacteria, stress, diet, smoking, environmental toxins or physical inactivity – even fat around the abdomen. Lingering inflammation can cause cell and tissue damage, and contribute to all kinds of conditions, such as immune imbalances, cardiovascular disease, gastrointestinal conditions, degenerative cognitive illnesses and cancer. Chronic inflammation can last for months, even years, if the immune system is not supported by lifestyle or dietary changes.

# when immunity overreacts

An efficient immune response protects against many conditions, while overactive immunity, underactive immunity or the wrong immune response can all cause havoc within the body, resulting in numerous health issues.

## autoimmunity

Autoimmune disorders occur when the body has become confused and starts to attack its own perfectly healthy cells and tissues. Why this happens is still unclear, but some theories suggest that certain viruses, prescription medication, chemicals and aspects of the diet (food sensitivities) might be responsible, or they may be the result of a genetic predisposition. There are more than 80 types of autoimmune disorders, including multiple sclerosis, coeliac (celiac) disease, rheumatoid arthritis, lupus erythematosus, psoriasis and type 1 diabetes – and the body can experience more than one.

## allergic reactions

Allergic reactions are a hypersensitive response to what is normally a harmless substance. Histamine is a chemical that causes these reactions and is found in the mast cells of connective tissue. It is released by the body when it experiences stress or comes into contact with a trigger. Inhaled allergens (pollen, dust mites, animal fur), medication (aspirin, penicillin, sulphur), food (fish, wheat, eggs, milk) and insect bites can all stimulate a reaction to varying degrees of severity.

During an allergic reaction, antibodies on mast cells attach to the invading allergen in an attempt to remove it, while the mast cell also releases histamine. This usually happens quickly, and the symptoms can range from mild – itching, burning or watery eyes, sneezing, rashes, congested sinuses and headaches – to the more severe – including spasms, stomach cramps and anaphylaxis, which involves difficulty breathing and can be life-threatening.

## how normal is it to get ill?

We now know that symptoms of a common cold are a sign that the immune system is at work trying to fend off the invading germs. It's perfectly normal to get a couple of colds a year, as the body is constantly exposed to pathogens. On the other hand, frequently coming down with colds, finding them hard to shake off or feeling run down can be signs that the immune system is under strain. This could be for several reasons – including stress, lack of exercise, poor diet or bad eating habits – so looking at lifestyle can help to identify potential causes or contributors.

**GP tip**

*To make a refreshing high-antioxidant, free-radical-fighting drink, squeeze five grapefruits or oranges into a jug, adding fizzy water. Low in sugar, high in vitamin C.*

### ▶ FOOD ALLERGIES

What makes food allergies different from intolerances or sensitivities is that the immune system gets heavily involved. It is triggered by particles or proteins in food that it interprets as dangerous, with reactions from mild to severe. The most common allergens are peanuts, nuts, milk, eggs, fish, shellfish, wheat and soy beans.

### ▶ HISTAMINE INTOLERANCE

Histamine intolerance is commonly caused by eating foods that contain histamine or that may trigger its release within the body. The immune system is not involved in this reaction, but the symptoms can be similar to a food allergy, which is why it can sometimes be hard to differentiate. Asthmatics can be particularly sensitive to histamine found in food, sometimes experiencing asthma attacks as a result.

Histamine-rich foods which are commonly problematic include alcohol (champagne and red wines are particularly high; white wine and beer are less so), chocolate, aged cheese, fermented foods (pickles, soy sauce, vinegar), avocados, unwashed dried fruit, aubergines and tinned and smoked fish. If you suspect you have this particular susceptibility, try to avoid these triggers.

### ▶ HAY FEVER

Hay fever has most of its fun in the warmer months of spring and summer, when trees and plants release more pollen. The allergic reaction occurs when the pollen is inhaled, triggering the release of histamine, which inflames the cells lining the nose and eyes. This causes symptoms like sneezing, coughing, itchy eyes, ears and throat, a blocked nose and fatigue.

### ▶ HIVES

Hives, or urticaria, occur when the body releases histamine, which causes plasma to leak from blood vessels in the skin. The skin responds by producing itchy, red welts that can appear anywhere on the body, including the face, lips, tongue or in the ears. They can last for hours or up to a day before fading and can be triggered by food, insect bites or stress.

*\* For serious reactions of any kind, always seek medical advice.*

*Combining antioxidant supplements is a great way to boost their effectiveness, helping build and support immunity. For example, quercetin, the hay fever-slayer, loves vitamin C, which increases its absorption.*

*My favourite natural anti-inflammatory cocktail is a combination of omega-3 oil, vitamins C and D and probiotics. And don't underestimate the power of exercise, which also helps calm this overreactive immune response.*

# *So what do we do?*

## ALL-STAR ANTIOXIDANTS

The following antioxidants are specifically involved in strengthening the immune defence and should be included as part of a balanced diet as there are some that the body can't synthesise. And when in doubt – as always, supplement.

## 1 PHYTOCHEMICALS

Phytochemicals are the pigments found in plants (fruit, vegetables, nuts, seeds, wholegrains and legumes) that not only protect them from UV rays and disease, but also give them their colour and flavour. As with plants, phytochemicals will also protect the body when eaten, reducing oxidative stress, inflammation and environmental aggressors. One of the largest group are the flavonoids. They are powerful antioxidants with anti-inflammatory, antibacterial, anti-allergic and other immune system benefits. Flavonoids are found in huge amounts in deeply coloured plant foods. Here are my three favourites:

### Anthocyanins

Defined as 'blue, violet or red flavonoid pigments found in plants', these are a triple threat with their antioxidant, anticarcinogenic and anti-inflammatory capabilities. They oversee the production of cytokines (chemicals that help immune regulation), reduce the risk of chronic diseases and prevent DNA cell damage:

▸ *Pomegranates, raspberries, strawberries, red peppers, purple grapes, plums, cherries, blueberries, blackberries.*

**GP** *tip*  *Fry, roast or bake quercetin-rich foods, or eat them raw. Just don't give them a hot bath, as quercetin is lost in boiling water.*

### Resveratrol

Resveratrol has been shown to modulate immune function, reduce inflammation and activate T cells, NK cells and macrophages (a type of phagocyte). Its antioxidant capabilities mean it is also able to regulate free radicals, preventing oxidative stress, and it has been shown to have antimicrobial properties, which supports a healthy intestinal microflora:

▸ *Grapes, red wine, peanuts (and peanut butter), soy, cocoa powder (very high), dark chocolate, blueberries, cranberries.*

### Quercetin

A powerful antioxidant and anti-inflammatory nutrient, quercetin is extremely effective for hay fever sufferers. It inhibits the release of histamine, reducing pro-inflammatory cytokines which would otherwise irritate the cell lining of the eyes, nose and throat:

▸ *Onions, red apples (high levels in the skin), honey, raspberries, red grapes, cherries, citrus fruits (oranges, lemons, limes), red leaf lettuce.*

**GP** *tip*  *A 40mg resveratrol supplement = 3 litres of red wine. I like wine, but that's A LOT. Just take the pill.*

**GP** *tip*

*Make home-made lollies by blitzing up natural live or nut yogurt with a big helping of mixed berries. If you don't have lolly moulds, freeze it in small cups with a spoon in the middle, which works as the stick. YUM.*

## 2 ANTIOXIDANT MINERALS
### Zinc

Zinc is incredibly important for several aspects of both the innate and adaptive immune systems. It assists in the development of their cells, as well as in the production of T and B cells and macrophages. It helps the immune system not to over-respond, managing levels of inflammation:

- ▸ *Plant foods: beans, nuts (almonds, cashews, hazelnuts, Brazil, walnuts), seeds (pumpkin, sunflower, flax, hemp, chia, pine nuts, wholegrains (oats, rye, buckwheat, brown rice), avocados, legumes (chickpeas, lentils, beans), berries (blueberries, raspberries, blackberries).*
- ▸ *Animal foods: red meat, shellfish (oysters, crab, prawns, mussels), poultry.*

### Selenium

Selenium protects against oxidative stress, which reduces inflammation. It has also been shown to help the body fight viral infections, as well as increase its resistance to them:

- ▸ *Brazil nuts (with exceptionally high levels), fish (tuna, halibut, sardines), shellfish (prawns), beef, turkey, chicken, cottage cheese, brown rice, eggs, beans, oats.*

**GP** *tip*

*One Brazil nut can have as much as double the recommended daily intake of selenium, making it easy to exceed this amount – so snack on them, don't gorge.*

## 3 ANTIOXIDANT VITAMINS
### Vitamin C

This antioxidant superhero protects the body against free radicals and regenerates fellow antioxidants such as vitamin E. It supports immunity by assisting in the production of leukocytes (lymphocytes and neutrophils particularly) and phagocytes:

- ▸ *Kiwi fruit, citrus fruit (orange, pomelo, grapefruit, clementine, lemon), berries (strawberries, blackberries, raspberries, blueberries), papaya, pineapple, cantaloupe melon, mango, Brussels sprouts, broccoli, cauliflower, cabbage, tomatoes, peas, kale and peppers.*

### Vitamin A and beta-carotene

Beta-carotene is a precursor to vitamin A and is the red, orange and yellow pigment found in fresh fruit and vegetables. Known as retinol, vitamin A stimulates the body's natural defences, has anti-inflammatory properties and helps regulate normal immune cell function. Vitamin A also helps to protect the structural and functional integrity of the respiratory and gastrointestinal tracts' mucosal lining:

- ▸ *Vitamin A: beef liver, dairy (ricotta cheese, natural live yogurt), oily fish.*
- ▸ *Beta-carotene: yellow, red and green leafy vegetables (spinach, carrot, sweet potato, peppers, pumpkin, butternut squash), mango, papaya, apricots.*

## Vitamin D

Vitamin D is not a vitamin, but actually a hormone produced by the body. It is one of the immune system's champion fighters. Modulating both innate and acquired immunity, it helps to activate the T cell response to infections and has been shown to reduce the risk of developing respiratory tract and autoimmune conditions.

The sun plays an important role in the body's synthesis of vitamin D during spring and summer. This is why vitamin D deficiencies are often seasonal, as reduced exposure to sunlight during the darker months typically results in commonplace illnesses like colds or flu.

The body synthesises 90 per cent of its vitamin D from contact with direct sunlight, although from September to early April this is hugely reduced for those who live in countries like the UK, so it's a good idea to take a supplement. Vitamin D is also found in:

▶ *Oily fish (mackerel, salmon, sardines, herring), egg yolks and whole milk.*

*Sun exposure before 10am without sunblock will give your body a hearty dose of vitamin D. Even as little as 15–20 minutes a day during the summer months can help top your levels up.*

## ESSENTIAL FATTY ACIDS – OMEGA-3

Amazing for the brain, hormone balancing, skin, hair and nail health, these nutrients could teach your children French, launch rockets from NASA, and, for all we know, explain what the hell bitcoin is – as well as being professional firefighters thanks to their anti-inflammatory capabilities. To say they are multi-talented is an understatement:

▶ *Oily fish (mackerel, salmon, sardines, herring), nuts (walnuts, almonds, hazelnuts, macadamia, pecans), seeds (sunflower, pumpkin, hemp, flax, chia).*

## BLOOD SUGAR BALANCE

What did I tell you? Sugar is mean. Imbalanced – specifically, elevated – blood sugar levels lead to chronic low-grade inflammation by trying to metabolise the excess glucose. To keep levels balanced, follow the GP principles on page 22 and see the Vital energy chapter (page 120).

## STRESS LEVELS

There is an undeniable link between stress and increased levels of inflammation, as the stress hormone cortisol is believed to interfere with immunity, stimulating the release of inflammatory-inducing chemicals. There are lots of ways to reduce stress in the body:

▶ *Magnesium supplements, exercise, lowering caffeine intake and breathing techniques. See the Hormones chapter on page 84.*

*Vegans and vegetarians should eat plenty of beta-carotene-rich foods, so the body can convert them into vitamin A.*

*Aim to eat 3–4 portions of oily fish a week – otherwise, supplement with omega-3 fish oils and algae oil for vegetarians and vegans.*

## MOVE YOUR LYMPH

The lymphatic system relies on muscle contraction for movement – the kind that occurs in hollow organs like the stomach and intestines and happens without us being aware of it. This is why physical inactivity can impact how efficiently the lymphatic system circulates, leading to it becoming sluggish and unable to distribute the immune cells needed to destroy pathogens throughout the body.

Being physically active – from just moving around to proper exercise – is really important, but other methods can also be effective:

▸ *Swim, shower or immerse the body in cold water on a regular basis.*
▸ *Dry-brush your skin or try lymphatic massage.*

## PROBIOTICS

The large intestine is home to trillions of beneficial bacteria, which have a monumental impact on the immune system and the regulation of inflammation. Not only can they reduce levels of unwanted bacteria by physically outnumbering them, but also by their very nature, they act as a kind of constant mild challenge to the immune system, making sure it is always low-level active and therefore better able to spring into action when pathogens invade. Probiotics are so important they should have their own TV show and merchandise:

▸ *Fermented foods: sauerkraut, kimchi, miso, tempeh, probiotic (live) yogurt, kefir, kombucha.*

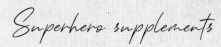

*Superhero supplements*

- Vitamin C & vitamin D
- Quercetin
- Probiotics
- N-acetyl cysteine
- Zinc
- Selenium
- Medicinal mushrooms – reishi, cordyceps, maitake

**GP** *tip*

*Take a multi-strain probiotic supplement, minimum 5–10 colony-forming units (CFU), for a month to support immunity, general health or if you've been prescribed antibiotics in the past 12 months.*

# 3/

## clean up
## *and* detoxify

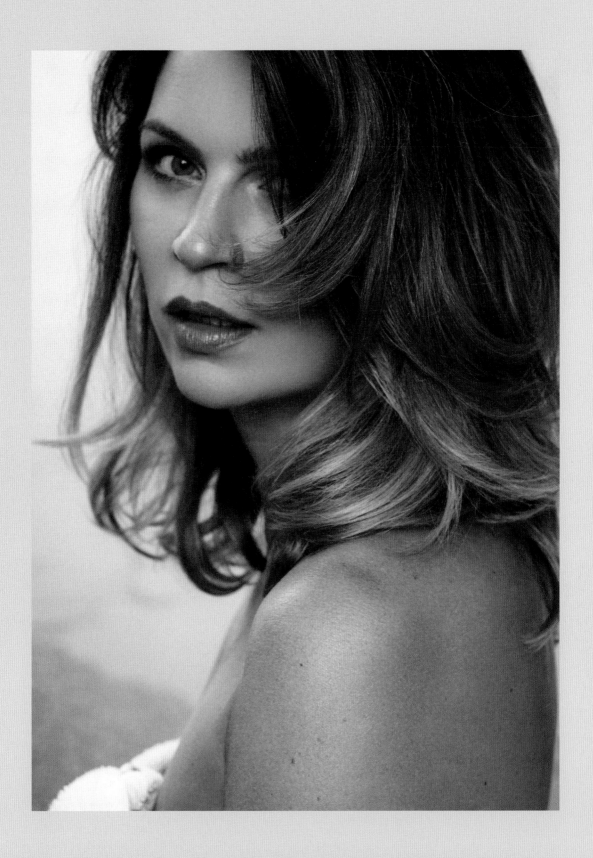

*do you* ...

☐ have temperamental skin?
☐ regularly feel sluggish and lethargic?
☐ often experience digestive complaints?
☐ feel caffeine has a negative effect on you?
☐ suffer from horrendous hangovers?

# meet the liver

The liver is a truly magnificent organ that performs over 500 jobs on a daily basis. It's the body's chemical filter, getting toxins ready for elimination through sweat, urine and the bowels in a multi-phase process.

Anything inhaled, eaten or absorbed passes through the liver, from the chemicals in the air we breathe, in the cosmetics and creams we put on our skin, in the products we use to clean our homes and in the water we drink, to the pesticides, additives and preservatives in our food, alcohol, cigarette smoke, medications and drugs.

And there's more. When hormones have done their work, they become redundant and have to be processed through the liver. It's the same with non-beneficial bacteria in the intestine. That is A LOT of work. The liver is an extraordinary, complex, highly intelligent organ that works relentlessly to keep the body in the best condition it can. And while we can't all live in air-purifying oxygen tents, anointing our skin only with organic baby emu oil, there are many ways to alleviate some of the strain.

GP
*tip*

*Help balance the sugar-spiking ways of alcohol or coffee with liver-loving snacks like nuts and seeds. The kind coated in chilli, matcha or dark chocolate are especially good with a cocktail. Supposedly. Not that'd I know, of course.*

# The stages of detoxification

Let's take the example of food. Once a mouthful of food has been chewed and swallowed, it makes its way to the stomach, where digestive enzymes get to work breaking everything down. The nutrients in what you've eaten are then absorbed through the intestinal wall from where they are distributed around the body. While all the helpful nutrients are busy getting to work, the body also needs to deal with everything that is either redundant, useless or harmful.

- **PHASE 1:** *The liver begins the process of making the fat-soluble toxins water-soluble, to prepare them for excretion. As these toxins are converted, free radicals are produced, which can damage the body's cells if they outnumber our antioxidants. On top of that, sometimes these intermediate molecules are more dangerous or reactive than the original substances.*

- **PHASE 2:** *Involves joining products from Phase 1 with nutrients like amino acids. This makes the toxins less reactive and also more water-soluble. They are now ready to be excreted in faeces, urine and sweat. Goodbye!*

Phase 1 and Phase 2 need to process at a similar speed to do their job as best they can. But this can easily be disrupted. Coffee, alcohol, cigarette smoke and chargrilled meat are just some of the triggers that increase Phase 1. This puts Phase 2 at risk of being unable to keep up with processing all the toxins, which can then escape into the body, causing havoc and attacking tissues. It's crucial for both phases to work at the same pace – so in theory, having a cup of coffee and increasing Phase 1 is not so terrible if you also focus on eating nutrient-rich foods, like pomegranate seeds, eggs or broccoli to give Phase 2 extra support.

## nutrients and the liver

Liver function is dependent on nutrients. These two are a match made in heaven, a love story for all ages. When the liver has used certain nutrients to prepare toxins for elimination, it uses others to escort them into the body's waste system. Nutrients are the body's facilitators.

If there are not enough nutrients in the diet, the body becomes unable to properly eliminate what it doesn't need or want and this can cause imbalances. Other systems responsible for energy levels, immunity or sleep – to name a few – also become negatively affected, because nutrients are diverted from their other roles in order to support an overloaded liver. This may lead to the body feeling weakened, sluggish and lethargic.

*Livers love lemon. Squeeze the juice into a glass of water and drink it through a straw, as it's acidic on the teeth. With hot water, keep it on the cool side, as heat tends to deteriorate the vitamin C content.*

*When possible, go organic with soft fruit like berries, as the pesticides on non-organic foods are harder to wash off and the liver will have to process them.*

# intestinal flora and the liver

Think of the intestine as a mini kingdom that is home to trillions of microbiomes – an ecosystem of intestinal flora designed to aid digestion, generate the 'happy' neurotransmitter serotonin, synthesise vitamins K and B12 and regulate around 70 per cent of the body's immunity. Having an imbalanced microbiota can compromise the intestinal barrier. Pathogens (microorganisms that can cause disease), toxins and foreign particles may then escape into the bloodstream, where they get picked up again by the portal vein and redirected back to the liver, giving it more work. Not good.

---

**SIGNS OF AN IMBALANCED MICROBIOTA**

▶ **Constipation**
Waste builds up in the colon and this leads to toxins and redundant hormones getting reabsorbed. They travel back to the liver, increasing its workload, and this can cause side effects like headaches, bloating, fatigue and skin problems.

▶ **Flatulence and bloating**
It's normal to have a balance of good and less-good bacteria in the intestine. However, if the less-good start to increase in number, they physically take the space of good bacteria, pushing them out. This is known as dysbiosis and can result in diarrhoea, constipation, flatulence and bloating.

---

# an unhappy liver upsets the skin

If the liver is overworked and struggling to get rid of impurities, they will find their way out through another route – and that can sometimes be the skin. While there can be many reasons for misbehaving skin, breakouts, inflammation and dryness are a clue that the liver is tired.

## a little note about caffeine

Caffeine is a stimulant found in food and drinks including coffee, black and green tea, chocolate and some fizzy drinks. Side effects like insomnia, headaches or feeling wired may be because the Phase 1 detoxification process is too slow and the liver is struggling to process caffeine. It may also be due to genetically derived slow enzyme function, where the body breaks down caffeine less efficiently. Equally, being able to knock back coffee late at night and go straight to sleep suggests Phase 1 is working too quickly – putting pressure on Phase 2.

*Don't drink caffeine on an empty stomach, as not only will it give you a sugar spike, it could leave you feeling wired. Instead, always have it with a snack or preferably with or after meals.*

# So what do we do?

There are lots of things we can do, big and small, like switching to clean beauty and personal-care brands, as well as non-toxic products that can be used to clean everything – face, body, hair, teeth, dishes, food, windows and the dog. Maybe don't try that at the same time though. When it comes to food and nutrients, there are so many options that will help the liver to flourish.

## 1 offenders in the home

### Plastics

Airtight plastic containers are standard in most kitchens, but the components they're made of, like the synthetic compound bisphenol A, can seep into food. Plastic bottles are particularly bad, especially during hot weather or when left in a hot car, as heat causes the chemicals in the bottle to leach into the liquid. The same goes for cling film or plastic wrap. Fatty foods like cheese and milk are particularly absorbent.

▸ *Use glass or stainless steel bottles, boxes or jars. Replace soft plastics with beeswax wraps, silicone lids or pouches.*

### Washing clothes

Many household brands use chemical fragrances that stick to clothes and can be toxic. Some of the worst culprits are optical brighteners, designed to make whites whiter, and dryer sheets that reduce static.

▸ *The skin is highly absorbent so opt for clean brand washing detergents.*

### Cleaning

We can all be a bit obsessive about creating a sterile environment, but that doesn't mean treating our homes like science laboratories. With the exception of the very elderly, small children, babies and people with low immunity, most of us have an immune system that can deal with standard bacteria exposure.

▸ *Swap abrasive chemical household products for gentler environmentally-friendly brands.*

### Kitchenware

Non-stick pots and pans contain chemicals that can get into food when heated. Non-stick is considered to be safe as long as the pan is not 'overheating', though – in other words, anything over 290°C (550°F). It turns out that it's incredibly easy to reach that temperature – preheating an empty non-stick pan for a couple of minutes or cooking on a high temperature for an extended period of time will exceed this.

▸ *Replace scratched or worn-out non-stick pans with stainless-steel, cast-iron, ceramic or enamel alternatives.*

**GP tip**

*Avoid heating food in plastic containers, as they may leach harmful compounds into what is about to be eaten. Instead, decant into non-plastic containers first. And always try to use a non-plastic, reusable bottle for water.*

*GP tip*

*A toxin-free DIY solution of one-part water and one-part vinegar is very effective for cleaning glass and stainless steel. Adding baking soda not only helps with tougher stains, but also reduces the vinegar smell, as does adding rosemary and lemon.*

# 2 skincare culprits

It's all about finding a balance that works and getting into the habit of checking ingredients to see if there are alternatives that can be used to reduce exposure. These are the ingredients to avoid – graded from 1 to 10 by the Environmental Working Group, with 10 being the worst.

| INGREDIENT + GRADING | WHAT IS IT? | WHERE TO LOOK OUT FOR IT |
|---|---|---|
| Parabens (propylparaben, butylparaben, isobutylparaben): *7–8* | A preservative used to extend the longevity of products. They are endocrine disruptors and can trigger hormone imbalances, sometimes leading to serious health problems. | Very commonly used in beauty products, especially those that are water-based like shampoo, conditioner, moisturiser, cleanser, sunscreen, deodorant, shaving gel, toothpaste and make-up. |
| Artificial fragrance: *8* | An artificial chemical listed as 'perfume', 'parfum' or 'fragrance' that can contain endocrine disruptors, carcinogens and irritants. It disturbs the immune system and can cause allergies. | A huge proportion of beauty products are scented – check for any indication that the product contains an artificial fragrance. |
| Sodium Lauryl Sulfate/ Sodium Laureth Sulfate (SLS/SLES): *8* | Foaming agents that give that 'clean' feel. They can irritate the skin and cause allergic reactions. | Anything that foams, e.g. body wash, toothpaste, foaming cleanser, shampoo, shaving cream. |
| Phythalates (DBP, DEHP, DEP): *7–10* | Added to plastic to keep it flexible and durable, they are endocrine disrupters and can contribute to the development of allergies. | Widely used in products like nail polish (especially those listed as chip-resistant), aftershave, fragrances and hair spray. |

| Oxybenzone: *6–8*<br>Octinoxate: *6*<br>Homosalate: *4*<br>Octisalate: *4*<br>Octocrylene: *3*<br>Avobenzone: *2* | Chemical filters used in some sunscreens. Endocrine disruptors and toxicant, they can trigger skin allergies and affect the thyroid. | Mass-market sunscreens, SPF lip balms, foundations and moisturisers. |
| --- | --- | --- |

*My gigantically tall body has a large surface area (I'm five foot eleven), while my face is small in comparison, so to moderate my chemical intake, I use organic skincare on my body and pretty much whatever I like on my face.*

## Deodorant and antiperspirant

The armpits are highly vulnerable (which is not a sentence you read every day). Lymph nodes sit right next to them under the skin and regular shaving can make the skin even more permeable. Synthetic antiperspirant formulas often contain chemicals that can disrupt hormone levels, such as parabens and aluminium, which is one of the worst offenders. The fragrance element is also chemical. There are no natural antiperspirants available yet, however, there are better alternatives.

## Cleanser and moisturiser

Try to steer clear of foaming products. Organic versions of these products are better whenever possible, especially for children.

▸ *Keep an eye out for what's in non-organic skincare. Some use effective ingredients, like vitamin C, which fight free radicals and help prevent UV damage, as well as hyaluronic acid, which plumps the skin. They may not be organic, but they have their benefits.*

## Sun cream

Most of the standard sunscreen brands are heaving with chemicals. We cover ourselves in this stuff, absorb it and then go splashing about in the sea, where it also gets into the water, damaging marine life. Chemical sunscreens gradually become ineffective when exposed to UV rays, which is why they need constant reapplication.

▸ *Mineral sunblock acts as a physical barrier to the sun's rays by sitting on the skin because the particles are too big to be absorbed. Some are quite thick to use, so try a few to find one that suits.*

*Natural, organic deodorants made with essential oils are much kinder to the skin and don't block pores.*

*A clean mineral sunscreen should only contain the actives zinc oxide and/or titanium dioxide, so always check.*

*Spray fragrances onto clothes and not the skin to reduce absorption (but still smell like a Disney princess).*

*GP tip*

*I find the build-up of natural oils in organic shampoo makes my hair a bit flat, so if I use non 'clean' hair products, I step out from under the shower and rinse my head upside down to minimise what I absorb through my body.*

## Shampoo and conditioner

Most average products contain a festival of chemicals which can cause skin irritation, particularly as they get all over our bodies in the shower. As well as stripping the hair's natural oils, many of the ingredients that conventional brands use to make hair look glossy, like silicone and polymers, do little to actually condition it.

▸ *The natural oils, butters and plant extracts in 'clean' products benefit the hair more, keeping it healthy and shiny.*

## Toothpaste

The inside of the mouth is more porous than the lips and the average tube of toothpaste contains chemicals like SLS and other agents believed to tackle plaque and gingivitis.

## Fragrance

Many fragrances contain artificial ingredients, like endocrine disruptors, which get into the body's system through the lungs, nose and skin. We are basically chemically spraying ourselves, even if it does smell good. Perhaps moderate how often you wear it.

## Lipstick

It's common for lipsticks, particularly red ones, to contain traces of petroleum, plasticisers and lead, which is a neurotoxin that affects the brain and nervous system. Lead has been removed from the paint we use on the walls of our homes, but we're still putting it on our faces. Quite weird when you think about it.

*GP tip*

*Using a clean toothpaste is non-negotiable for me. My general rule is, if it can't be eaten, don't brush your teeth with it.*

*GP tip*

*I love occasionally wearing red lipstick, but as the lips are highly absorbent, I usually opt for a tinted organic lip balm.*

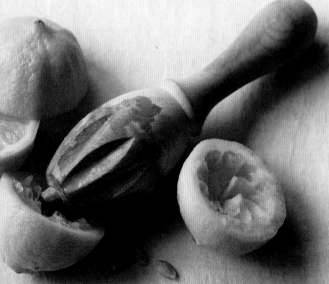

*3 shop for the liver*

### ORGANIC VERSUS NON-ORGANIC

There is a huge debate about organic versus non-organic and it can be hard to decide to what degree we should change our shopping habits. Organic produce is expensive and tends not to last, which is hard when most people don't have the time to shop every day. So how do we make it work for us?

## Meat, fish, eggs and dairy

The problem with eating non-organic meat, fish, eggs and dairy is the increased probability of consuming what these animals may have been exposed to. They tend to be fed on pesticide-rich grains, given hormones to grow faster or produce more milk and antibiotics to get rid of infections. What they've had in their systems, we get into ours when we eat them.

## Fruit and vegetables

While there's no denying the appeal of fat, juicy GMO cherries in the middle of winter, it would be better – finances permitting – to include as much organic produce in the diet as possible. Those who have ever eaten a greasy apple might be interested to know that this is a result of a chemical fertiliser containing fat, which sticks to the skin so that it can't be washed off by rain or through watering. Eww. Organic farming does not permit the use of pesticides, synthetic fertilisers or chemicals, so while it may be demoralising to watch organic carrots shrivelling before your eyes because their shelf life is so much shorter, there are ways to create a happy medium.

*You can go non-organic with harder fruit and vegetables, scrubbing the ones where the skin is eaten with a brush and a specially formulated fruit-and-vegetable wash (just running them under water won't properly clean them).*

# 4 the liver superheroes

## SULPHUROUS FOODS

Sulphurous foods are generally very beneficial for the liver, including an anti-inflammatory effect. Pungent, yes – but think of the smile it'll put on the liver's face... if it had a face.

## Cruciferous vegetables

Not all heroes wear capes. Some of them come with overlapping leaves instead. The superior powers of cruciferous vegetables are in its glucosinolates – compounds containing sulforaphane, which is particularly good at neutralising the effects of toxins. They are top of the class in supporting Phase 1, but even more so with Phase 2.

▸ *Cabbages, cauliflower, kale, broccoli, Brussels sprouts, kale, bok choy.*

## The allium family

Allicin is a sulphuric compound found in foods like garlic, leeks and onions and is what gives them their strong taste and odour. It supports Phase 2 of the liver's detoxification process.

▸ *Onion, garlic, chives, shallots, leeks.*

## Eggs

Aside from being high in protein and healthy fats, eggs are a sulphurous food that also support Phase 2 detoxification. They contain the amino acids which contribute to the production of glutathione, the powerful antioxidant that is present throughout the body and protects cells against the potential damage of free radicals.

*Important sulphur knowledge – let garlic sit for a few minutes after crushing or grating to allow the beneficial compounds to activate. And if you struggle to digest eggs, try taking a digestive enzyme as you eat them.*

## Berries and their friends

Berries contain beneficial plant chemicals called anthocyanins, which is what gives them their typically red, blue and purple colour. Not only are anthocyanins good for the brain and memory, they also happen to be highly potent antioxidants that protect against cell damage. Berries also contain the nutrient ellagic acid, which has antioxidant and antiviral properties and scavenges and destroys free radicals, regulating Phase 1 and 2 enzyme production and moderating inflammation.

▸ *Cherries, pomegranates, strawberries, blueberries, cherries, blackberries, raspberries, blackcurrants, red grapes, pomegranates, cranberries.*

## Essential fatty acids

Apart from being high in essential fatty acids, avocado is one of the few foods to contain glutathione, plus it also helps to detoxify our bodies from heavy metals. Nuts, seeds and oily fish like salmon, sardines and mackerel are all rich in omega-3 fatty acids, which assist in reducing inflammation and prevent oxidative stress, making them essential for optimal liver function. Nuts also contain vitamin E and other antioxidants, and Brazil nuts are packed with selenium, which the liver needs in high levels to help it produce glutathione.

▸ *Oily fish (salmon, mackerel, sardines, herring), nuts (Brazil, cashew, macadamia, almond, walnut, hazelnut), seeds (pumpkin, sunflower, chia, flax, hemp), avocado.*

## Probiotics

Fermented foods are loaded with healthy probiotic bacteria, which have been shown to improve toxin elimination. Some probiotic bacteria work by reducing the amount of toxins the intestine absorbs, so that fewer are sent to the liver. Probiotic-rich foods can help maintain a healthy intestinal lining, preventing impurities from breaking through and entering the bloodstream, as well as supporting efficient digestion and elimination processes.

▸ *Natural live yogurt, sauerkraut, kimchi, kombucha, kefir, tofu, miso, tempeh.*

## Citrus fruit

Citrus fruit contains numerous beneficial compounds, such as flavonoids, vitamins (particularly vitamin C), carotenoids, essential oils, minerals and dietary fibre. These compounds have been proven to have a protective effect on the liver, especially when it's under stress with excessive alcohol consumption.

▸ *Lemons, oranges, grapefruits, limes, tangerines, clementines, satsumas, yuzu.*

*Adding freshly squeezed lemon juice to slightly cooled green tea makes it even more delicious and takes away the bitterness that can put some people off – plus, vitamin C helps increase the absorption of catechins.*

*Give avocado new life by turning it into... ice cream. Blend 2 avocados, 1 can of coconut milk, 5 tablespoons of agave, 4 tablespoons of lime juice, 2 teaspoons of lime zest and 3 tablespoons of water – and freeze. Easy.*

# a little note about red wine

Red wine contains anthocyanins and ellagic acid, both of which we have now established are good for the body. Let's not forget the sugar content and the fact that alcohol has an inflammatory effect – but, hurray and thank you, life.

### Turmeric (curcumin)

The curcumin in this brightly coloured spice is an all-round anti-inflammatory nutrient that assists the liver in a lot of different ways, supporting Phase 2 detoxification and boosting levels of glutathione. It has also been shown to protect the liver against damage from chemicals and support digestion.

### Green tea (catechins)

Green tea is packed with polyphenols, which are highly effective antioxidants, the most important of which are catechins. These have been shown to increase the performance of detoxification enzymes in the liver by binding to toxic compounds. In fact, studies have shown that as few as three cups of green tea a day could reduce the risk of breast cancer.

### Wheatgrass

Iron. Magnesium. Antioxidants. Chlorophyll. Amino acids. Calcium. Vitamins A, C and E. Behold the considerable roll call of goodness that makes up wheatgrass. This stuff is so healthy, it's ridiculous.

*Start small with half a shot of fresh wheatgrass and build up slowly. If you find the flavour too strong, add the more gentle-tasting organic wheatgrass powder to smoothies or juices.*

*Turmeric in powder form needs to be mixed with a fat to help the body absorb it more efficiently. Melt a teaspoon of coconut oil, mix it with the turmeric powder into a paste and then add it to hot milk, soup or curry.*

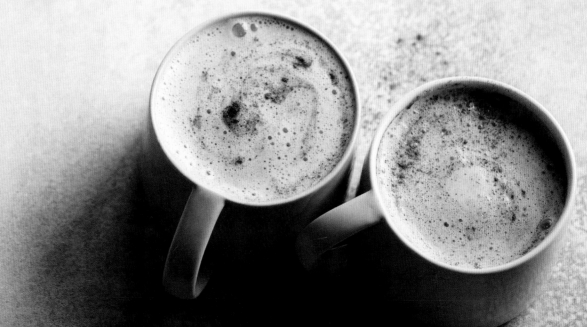

## HOW TO HANDLE A HANGOVER

That brutal morning of regret when it was all so hilarious the night before. Hangovers are a mixture of dehydration and symptoms often induced by pressure on the liver – headaches, nausea, exhaustion, general grumpiness. As alcohol is broken down, potentially harmful by-products are produced. To get rid of them, the body will declare a state of emergency and prioritise the liver. Nutrients normally used for digestion and energy production will rush to the liver's aid, focussing less on their other jobs, to help the liver flush the alcohol out, but inevitably making the body feel even worse in the process.

A breakfast of the right food can help kick hangovers into touch. Meal composition is vital to help balance blood sugar levels and prevent any further energy dips or mood swings throughout the day. Unfortunately, a slice of toast with honey or a pastry won't make the grade. Protein is an important macronutrient the body needs to help it recover, as it contains the amino acids to support liver detoxification.

### Pick and mix saviour breakfast

Fantasising over a fry-up or last night's pizza for breakfast is a desert mirage that is not to be trusted. What the body needs is a combination of proteins and carbs, so here is a table with some ideas to help combat the horror:

| PROTEIN | CARBOHYDRATE |
|---|---|
| 1–2 slices smoked salmon | 110g (4oz) berries |
| 2 eggs | 1–2 slices dark rye / pumpernickel bread (or gluten-free option) |
| 3 slices turkey breast | 3 oatcakes or rye crackers |
| 120g (4oz) live dairy / coconut / nut yogurt | 40g (1½oz) muesli / low-sugar granola |
| Small handful of nuts / seeds | 40g (1½oz) porridge oats |
| 2–3 tablespoons nut butter | 2–3 brown rice / buckwheat / almond flour pancakes |
| 250ml (9fl oz) nut milk | 40g (1½oz) bran flakes / shredded wheat |

*I could recommend going for a run with hangovers – if I were cruel and unusual – but instead I suggest a detoxifying bath with magnesium flakes, which will also help with much-needed sleep.*

## Crisis smoothie

If there's not enough time for a proper breakfast, let's keep things simple – rough measurements and just put it all in a blender.

- Small handful of mixed nuts and seeds
- Half an avocado
- Handful of mixed berries
- Tablespoon of coconut oil
- Mixed superfood powder (acai, raspberry, blueberry, bilberry, goji, cherry)

- Half a banana
- 1–2 scoops of protein powder or half a pot of plain live yogurt (protein is key – don't leave it out).
- Add oat or nut milk of your choosing.

## Emergency rehydration

For those who have woken up with a mouth dryer than a sandpit, here are the best things to start your day with.

▸ *Fresh green juice*
*Use a mixture of cruciferous vegetables, like broccoli or kale, plus anything else green that is to hand – spinach, cucumber or celery. Sweeten it with a green apple and add lemon juice.*

▸ *Diluted coconut water or fruit juice*
*Water is the best thing to rehydrate with, but the body may crave something sweeter and a little more substantial, so try mixing it with coconut water or fruit juice. Don't add more than a third of a glass, though, as they're pretty sugar-heavy and can cause a blood sugar spike and then a drop, which will be more savage than normal.*

▸ *Kombucha*
*This delicious fermented drink is fantastic at settling a disagreeable hangover stomach, as it's full of probiotics, which will help rebalance the intestine flora, supporting the liver flush out any remaining impurities.*

## HELP ME!!!!! hot drinks

If you have reached the stage where you're crying and you want your mother, these help.

▸ *Turmeric / matcha latte*
· ½ teaspoon of turmeric or matcha powder.
· Heated nut or oat milk.
· A squeeze of agave.

▸ *Green / matcha tea*
*Use a teabag and boiling water. Obvious, yes, but not to those who are hungover.*

## Superhero supplements

- Choline
- Curcumin
- L-methionine
- N-acetyl cysteine
- Alpha-lipoid acid
- Green superfoods powder
- Selenium
- Artichoke extract

# 4/

## sleep *and* relaxation

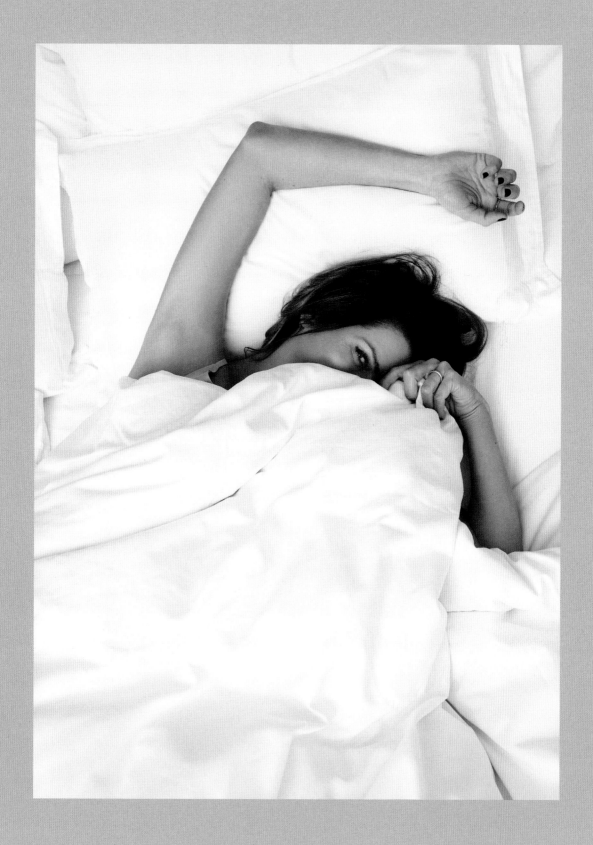

- [ ] often wake up feeling tired?
- [ ] have sugar cravings throughout the day?
- [ ] feel hungry before you go to bed?
- [ ] wake up in the night and find it hard to fall back to sleep again?
- [ ] drink alcohol more than three times a week?

# why do we need sleep?

A good night's sleep is a thing of beauty. The body does a lot when we're asleep – everything from growing muscle, repairing damaged tissue and producing hormones to supporting the cardiovascular system and metabolism. The brain also regroups and resets in myriad ways. The better the body sleeps, the more efficiently all of this happens.

When we're asleep, the brain gets to work flushing out waste products and redundant cells that accumulate during the course of the day. The brain's prefrontal cortex, which is in charge of decision-making, is constantly active during waking hours. Thinking is what it does all day, every day, even during supposed periods of relaxation. That's one of the many reasons why good sleep is so crucial, because it's the only time the outrageously busy prefrontal cortex actually gets to rest.

One of sleep's most important roles is allowing the brain to process and consolidate memories from the day's experiences, wiring and firing the neural pathways it needs for thinking and learning. When sleep is disrupted, it can result in poor concentration, bad moods, a very sketchy memory and an inability to take in new information. Misery.

**GP tip**

*My latest evening snack discovery is tryptophan-rich roasted chickpeas instead of crisps or popcorn. In short: drain, rinse, cover in oil and salt, roast for 20–30 minutes on 200°C (400°F), gas mark 6, turning occasionally. Crunch down with Netflix.*

# a closer look at the sleep cycle

Don't be fooled into thinking that being asleep is just a state of unconsciousness. On the contrary. A healthy sleep cycle is made up of four stages, which last around 90 minutes and are repeated several times over the course of a night.

**STAGE ONE:**
As the body starts to fall asleep, the first stage of the cycle begins with what is known as 'non-rapid eye movement' (non-REM) sleep. The body is drifting off, but hasn't completely relaxed during this light sleep phase, which usually lasts around 1 to 5 minutes.

**STAGE TWO:**
The body's temperature now starts to drop, triggering blood pressure, heart rate and breathing to slow down and muscles to relax. Stage two lasts around 25 minutes and gets longer with every repetition of the cycle. It is still non-REM sleep, so no dreams about having to retake exams in a house of cheese – yet.

**STAGE THREE:**
It is now time to enter deep sleep, which is still non-REM, but the critical part of the cycle for rebuilding muscle and tissue, strengthening immunity, balancing energy and releasing hormones. While it's true this phase gets shorter with age, being woken from it doesn't get easier. Everybody knows that groggy feeling that comes with being woken in the night and that can take up to an hour to subside.

**STAGE FOUR:**
The famous 'rapid eye movement' (REM) part of the cycle, where the brain likes to get creative. Dream sleep is when the brain sorts through different experiences and emotions, storing memories, learning and regulating mood. This phase can last from anything between 20–60 minutes.

**STAGES THREE** and **FOUR** are the most important phases of the cycle, as they're the ones where most of the physical and psychological work takes place. The amount of sleep a person needs tends to vary, as some are capable of functioning perfectly well on only a handful of hours. In an ideal world, getting seven to nine hours of proper sleep is enough time to complete a few rounds of the sleep cycle so that the body wakes feeling adequately rested.

Alas, the modern world with its noise, lights and screens has put a dent in that plan, with the average person only managing six and a half hours a night. Ongoing poor sleep will then increase the likelihood of turning to caffeine to feel awake in the day and then alcohol or sleep medication to unwind in the evening. All this does is disrupt what is actually a simple and very natural process for the body, run by the highly intelligent circadian rhythm.

# Circadian rhythm

The circadian rhythm is an internal clock within the brain, which synchronises with the body's environment to trigger when it's time to sleep and when it's time to wake up. This biological system responds to changes in light because the body is pre-programmed to align its activity with that of the sun. Think back to a time when there was no artificial light – humans would wake at sunrise and retire when it got dark because they were no longer able to hunt, forage or perform any practical tasks. Things have moved on since then, and while we can now go to a 24-hour shop instead of having to wrestle an antelope to the ground for dinner, daylight and darkness still play key roles in regulating the body's temperature, metabolism and the release of hormones.

The circadian rhythm is run by the part of the brain known as the hypothalamus. This region is responsible for maintaining the body's homeostasis, or internal balance.

In order to wake the body in the morning, the eye's optic nerve sends a signal to the hypothalamus as soon as it senses light, kick-starting a TIME TO GET UP, IT'S MORNING sequence. The hypothalamus sends a message to raise the body's temperature, make the heart rate and blood pressure get a bit of wind in their sails and to stop the brain producing the sleepy chemical, melatonin. The

body enters a more conscious state, with memory, concentration and alertness coming back to life. Sleep has now ended. Good morning.

Conversely, when it starts to get dark at night, the hypothalamus picks up on the decreasing natural light and sends out a different set of instructions. It tells the body it feels sleepy, signalling for its core temperature to drop and the release of melatonin. Drowsiness begins and... can't quite remember where we... so tired... good ni... zzzzz.

It's all a bit more complicated now. Many of us stay up late, surrounded by artificial lighting, smartphones, TVs and laptops, all beaming their stimulating glow in our faces. Those biological systems that regulate sleep end up all over the shop, which has a knock-on effect, health-wise, as the body is unable to fulfil its night-time duties effectively. Constantly waking up feeling exhausted is hard enough, but these disruptions can go deeper.

# hormones love sleep

There are several hormones that rely on the circadian rhythm and the body sleeping to maintain their regulation and metabolism. When their work is thrown off by lack of sleep, the consequences are far more widespread than just feeling tired and needing to down gallons of coffee. Here are a handful of examples of how some of the body's key hormones can be disrupted:

| | |
|---|---|
| **GROWTH HORMONE** | Essential for growth and tissue repair, levels increase during sleep. Disrupted sleep can suppress production and cell regeneration. |
| **GHRELIN** | Responsible for stimulating the appetite. Poor sleep can cause spikes, which leads to cravings. |
| **LEPTIN** | Responsible for controlling the appetite. Levels drop with poor sleep and the body feels less full, encouraging it to eat. |
| **MELATONIN** | Crucial to regulating sleep by telling the body when it's time to go to bed. Its levels are increased at night, triggered to release by the reduction in daylight. Stress compromises production and stimulates wakefulness. |
| **CORTISOL** | Levels peak just before waking, making us feel hungry and alert. Bad sleep triggers more cortisol in the day, making the body overstimulated at night. |
| **INSULIN** | Balances blood sugar by managing glucose released through food. Bad sleep disrupts production and regulation, resulting in low energy and cravings. |

# tired bodies make bad choices

Research from the National Sleep Foundation has shown that some people who sleep badly can consume up to 300 more calories and twice as much fat in a day as someone who averages a solid eight hours. It's a nightmare, but it's true – bad sleep can make you gain weight.

A sleep-deprived body is more likely to crave a hit of sugary food to give it that quick energy boost, especially during the afternoon. Unfortunately, the body releases less insulin after eating when it's tired, leaving blood sugar spikes unmanaged. Instead, it releases more cortisol and adrenaline, its stress hormones, in an effort to stay awake by trying to increase alertness. This further compromises insulin levels, leaving a whole load of glucose hanging around in the bloodstream, causing chaos with blood sugar balance, energy levels and, inevitably, appetite.

It's also true that feeling hungry late at night may mean that the last meal consumed was not balanced with enough protein or that the gap between dinner and sleep was too long, causing blood sugar levels to drop. This can then disrupt the ease with which the body falls asleep, so eating regularly and eating well have an enormous positive impact.

*Timing and composition are key. Eating regular, balanced meals throughout the day, ending with a light supper that has more protein and vegetables than refined carbs delivers constant and steady blood sugar levels. Your prize is a better night's sleep.*

# stress cycle and sleep

It is a natural part of the circadian rhythm to release cortisol in the morning, which alerts the body that it's time to wake up. As the day progresses, cortisol levels gradually start to decline, reaching their lowest point in the evening, when the body begins to release melatonin, helping it prepare for sleep. However, stress can turn all of this upside down by continually releasing cortisol, which can then in turn suppress the secretion of melatonin, especially if feelings of stress continue into the evening. Falling asleep becomes much more of a challenge with all these hormone levels out of whack – as does falling asleep again after waking in the night. Stress and sleep are a match made in hell.

# alcohol and sleep

Having a few drinks before bed can seem like a good idea, but the sedative effect of alcohol is deceptive. Sleep might come easily to begin with, but the sugar in the alcohol will then disrupt blood sugar balance, triggering the body to keep waking up. It also prevents REM sleep, the most important part of the sleep cycle for emotional, mental and physical health. This is known as 'REM sleep rebound' and occurs after the liver and kidneys have worked to process all the alcohol, which is a job in itself. The brain then decides it can now catch up on the much-needed REM sleep, which typically involves weirdly vivid dreams towards the end of the sleep cycle over a shorter period of time. The body wakes up exhausted and regretting all that wine.

Alcohol is, of course, also a diuretic, increasing the body's need to use the bathroom in the night and causing it to sweat. All this and there's a thumping dehydration headache and groggy feeling waiting to join the party when morning comes. The disrupted sleep stages will of course only make it harder for the body to recover. Hangovers are not here to make friends.

*On a boozy night, alternating glasses of water and alcohol is a better option than downing water before bed, reducing the need for a night-time pee. Plus you might not drink as much alcohol and come up (almost) smiling the next day.*

# So what do we do?

There may be many reasons why sleep is a problem. The good news is, there are just as many helpful tips that can help to improve it.

## THE THREE WONDER NUTRIENTS FOR SLEEP

Magnesium, tryptophan and L-theanine are my favourite nutrients when it comes to improving sleep. Magnesium is the most important, as it's directly responsible for relaxing the body, but combining it with the other nutrients will increase the chances of a restful night's sleep.

## 1 MAGNESIUM

Magnesium is known as nature's relaxant. It reduces anxiety, muscle spasms, high blood pressure and has an amazing effect on sleep. Magnesium deficiency is incredibly common, with up to 80 per cent of the UK population not having enough in their diet. Increasing magnesium improves sleep onset, length, quality and feeling refreshed in the morning. The issue is that aside from aiding sleep, the body uses a huge amount of magnesium for various other jobs. If sleep deprivation is an ongoing issue, trying to source it through diet alone would require eating enormous quantities of dark leafy greens to even touch the sides of the amount needed to help. There are other ways to increase levels of magnesium in the body in addition to food.

- *Magnesium supplements – take them any time, but preferably mid-afternoon, as they will start to relax the body for the evening.*
- *Magnesium bath flakes – soak in them for at least 20 minutes.*
- *Magnesium-rich food – dark leafy greens (kale, cavolo nero, chard), seeds (pumpkin, flax, chia), nuts, beans, chickpeas, lentils, grains (quinoa, buckwheat), dark chocolate (65–70 per cent cocoa).*

*Magnesium chloride flakes tend to be the most effective when it comes to sleep, plus they're cleaner and superior in quality.*

*Magnesium glycinate or malate are the best combinations to take, as they are easily absorbed by the body. Magnesium citrate has a mild laxative effect, so beneficial if constipation is an issue. Consider magnesium in powder form, as it may be easier to take a higher dose than capsules.*

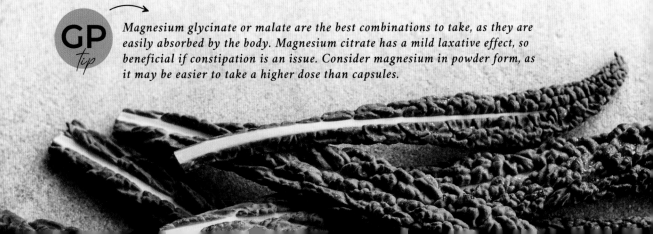

## 2 TRYPTOPHAN

Tryptophan is an amino acid found within protein. It is known for its ability to increase the production of serotonin (the happy and calming neurotransmitter in the brain) and assist in the body's ability to not only fall asleep but stay asleep:

► *Dairy products, peanuts, pumpkin and sesame seeds, poultry and eggs.*

## 3 L-THEANINE

This amino acid encourages relaxation and the ability to sleep by boosting levels of GABA, serotonin and dopamine (neurotransmitters in the brain that have a soothing effect). It's also known to reduce stress and anxiety:

► *Tea leaves (which also contain caffeine, so unless the tea is decaffeinated, supplement form may prove to be a better option. Go for a dose that is 200mg, or more).*

*Eat a couple of spoonfuls of cottage cheese or live yogurt, or a few slices of turkey or chicken before going to bed. These super-quick and convenient protein snacks require no preparation and the tryptophan will help induce sleepiness.*

## BALANCE BLOOD SUGAR LEVELS

Making sure blood sugar levels are balanced throughout the day will help maintain a healthy pattern that allows the body to follow its natural course towards falling asleep at night. I recommend these three principles:

► *Eating regularly – every 3–4 hours.*
► *Always eat when peckish, not starving.*
► *Include protein with every meal or snack.*

## KEEP AN EYE ON CAFFEINE

The body's ability to break down caffeine is largely genetic. Some people can process it through their livers much more quickly and efficiently than others. Everybody knows their own response to caffeine, so managing it is a personal thing. However, here are some ways to reduce caffeine intake:

► *Herbal teas, specifically chamomile. Many brands also make sleep blends.*
► *Turmeric latte – add black pepper and a teaspoon of coconut oil.*
► *Chicory coffee – roasted and grounded, these beans are not dissimilar to coffee.*

## WHAT ABOUT DINNER?

It's very important for the evening meal to be well composed, so not too high in carbs like rice, potatoes and pasta, and always including plenty of protein (lean meat, dairy, eggs, fish, nuts, lentils, beans) and non-starchy vegetables (broccoli, kale, asparagus, spinach). Low-fibre carbohydrates will spike the blood sugar levels, disrupting sleep, so give those a swerve. And without sounding like the place where fun goes to die, I would advise keeping an eye on sugary puddings and one too many glasses of wine, both of which can throw a spanner in the blood sugar works.

► *Switch to healthy puddings, such as fresh fruit or home-made ice cream made of yogurt and berries. A couple of squares of dark chocolate is not terrible either.*

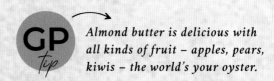

*Almond butter is delicious with all kinds of fruit – apples, pears, kiwis – the world's your oyster.*

## BREAK BAD BEDTIME HABITS

Aside from the supplements and food recommendations, I usually make practical suggestions to clients around sleep hygiene that are simple to implement:

### ▸ Notebook

Busy minds keep exhausted bodies awake. Having a notebook by the bed can help calm racing thoughts. Jotting down 'to-do' lists at 3am is better than ruminating on them.

### ▸ Temperature

The body's core temperature needs to drop before it can fall asleep and then stay asleep, so ensure that there is a window open with fresh air coming in and that the room is around 18°C (64°F).

### ▸ Regularity

Form a habit. Going to bed and waking up at the same time every day (including weekends – sorry) will really help create a rhythm for the body. Any kind of repeated night-time ritual, like having a bath, reading or listening to soothing music, reinforces this.

### ▸ Exercise

As little as 10 minutes of aerobic exercise a day (anything from walking to cycling to taking a HIIT class) can radically improve sleep quality. Some gentle forms of yoga or Pilates can actually encourage relaxation, but try to avoid anything too energetic just before bed.

### ▸ Screens

Avoid screen time at bedtime. The blue light that smartphones, computers and tablets emit can cause havoc with sleep, deceiving our brains into thinking it's daytime. As a result, the melatonin we need doesn't get released and the circadian rhythm gets knocked off track. Ideally, stop using devices at least one hour before bed, put them onto night mode or buy blue-light-blocking glasses.

**GP tip**

*A lovely, fragrant, decaffeinated alternative to teas like Earl Grey and English Breakfast is Red Bush (Roiboos). Not only can you add milk, but it tastes very similar to regular tea.*

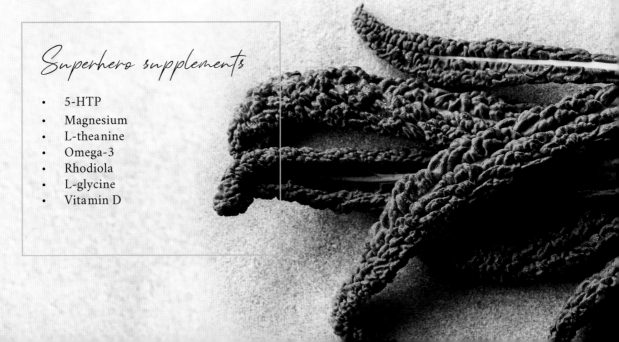

## Superhero supplements

- 5-HTP
- Magnesium
- L-theanine
- Omega-3
- Rhodiola
- L-glycine
- Vitamin D

# 5/

# digestion *and* absorption

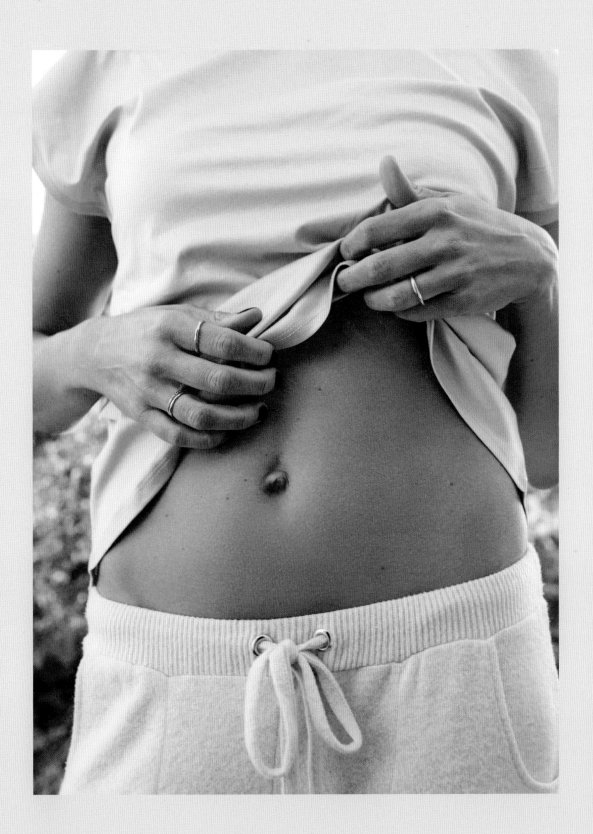

# meet the digestive system

The digestive system is complex and intriguing, playing a critical role in many aspects of the body's health. It is made up of the gastrointestinal tract, a long continuous tube that starts at the mouth, travels down the oesophagus, through the stomach, small intestine and large intestine before finishing at the anus.

The tongue, teeth and salivary glands are all accessory components that begin the initial phase of breaking down and digesting food. They are followed later by the liver, gallbladder and pancreas, which all play a multitude of important roles in the digestion and absorption of nutrients. This is very much a team effort, with each structure being relied on to get the job done before passing it on like a baton in a relay.

## digestion: step by step

### MOUTH
### – where it begins

As soon as we even start to think about food, the brain sends signals to the mouth to prepare by producing saliva and the enzyme salivary amylase. Once we eat a mouthful of food, the mechanical breakdown begins with the teeth chewing it up. This not only makes the food easier to swallow, but also increases its surface area, which will make it quicker for digestive chemicals and enzymes to do their job later in the process. At the same time, salivary amylase gets to work on the chemical breakdown of carbohydrates and starches specifically.

## OESOPHAGUS
### – a brief encounter
The oesophagus is the tube that connects the mouth and stomach. Peristalsis, a wave-like contraction of muscles, swiftly pushes swallowed food down the oesophagus and into the stomach. The stomach opens to receive it and then quickly shuts again until the next mouthful is ready to be received.

## STOMACH
### – the breakdown
The stomach serves as a waiting room, where digestion continues, but over an extended period of time. Gastric acid, secreted by the cells in the stomach lining, start breaking down fats and converting proteins into amino acids. Vitamin B12 is also separated from protein in our food and attached to another protein, which will help its absorption later in the small intestine. In the stomach, food, saliva and gastric acid are churned together, into a kind of pulp called chyme. During this process, any bacteria that may have smuggled their way in are killed off by the acidic juices. The chyme is then gradually released into the duodenum, the first part of the small intestine.

## SMALL INTESTINE
### – majorly absorbing
The small intestine is actually the longest part of the gastrointestinal tract, measuring between 3 and 5 metres (10 and 16 feet). The lining of this folded organ is covered in thousands of minute finger-like structures, like the bristles of a brush, called villi. Each individual villus is covered in hundreds of even smaller projections called microvilli – which maximises the surface area of the small intestine and increases its capacity to absorb nutrients. This surface is very thin, allowing easy absorption into the villi's capillaries so nutrients, like simple sugars, amino acids, water-soluble vitamins and

minerals, can be transported via the blood to the liver. Fats and fat-soluble vitamins are not water soluble, so cannot be carried via the blood. Instead, they are transported across the surface of the microvilli into lymphatic capillaries called lacteals. Through this private transportation system, fats are carried via the lymphatic system to the liver, where they are either processed for multiple jobs or stored.

The small intestine and pancreas secrete digestive enzymes, which continue the breakdown of the fats, proteins and carbohydrates in the chyme into nutrients. These are then absorbed, along with any water. The small intestine also secretes mucus, which works with pancreatic enzymes to neutralise the acidic contents of the chyme, preventing any damage to its unprotected lining.

Simultaneously, the liver produces bile, which is transferred via the gallbladder directly into the small intestine. Bile is particularly important for the digestion and absorption of fats and fat-soluble vitamins. Further waves of peristalsis mix all these secretions with the chyme, moving on whatever cannot be digested or absorbed (like insoluble fibre) to the large intestine as waste.

## LARGE INTESTINE
### – and now, the end is near
The large intestine or colon marks the final stage of digestion. Water is reabsorbed through the lining of the large intestine, along with remaining nutrients like the B vitamins, vitamin K, potassium and magnesium, while a large community of friendly bacteria get to work breaking down (or fermenting) any undigested food or indigestible fibres (dietary fibre). Only waste and whatever dietary fibre cannot be broken down is left. It moves through the lower part of the large intestine (the bowel) and is then stored there until excretion.

*Check your stomach acid levels by adding ¼ teaspoon of bicarbonate of soda to half a glass of water and drink on an empty stomach. You will burp after 3–4 minutes if levels are fine, while no reaction means levels are low.*

# magnificent microbiota

The digestive tract, specifically the intestine, is home to trillions of bacteria and other organisms, otherwise known as the intestinal microbiota. These microorganisms are a diverse community of good, less good, fine, quite bad, really quite bad and dial 999 bacteria. In order to maintain homeostasis, there needs to be a healthy balance between the beneficial and less beneficial kind.

The intestine is also where up to 70 per cent of the body's immune system lives. There are many things that can disrupt the harmony – stress, alcohol, bad sleep, diet, antibiotics – and when equilibrium is disturbed it causes imbalances (dysbiosis), with symptoms like bloating, flatulence, diarrhoea and constipation.

## what does our intestinal microbiota actually do?

▸ The gastrointestinal lining houses an elaborate network of 100 million neurons, often referred to as the 'second brain', which communicates with the central nervous system. The balance of the microbiota can directly influence our emotions, moods and general health.

▸ Microbiota ferment and feed on any remaining proteins, fibres, starches, or sugars in the large intestine and they synthesise essential nutrients like vitamin K and B vitamins.

▸ Around 95 per cent of serotonin (the body's 'happy neurotransmitter') comes from the cells lining the digestive tract and plays an integral role in appetite, digestion, sleep, memory and mental health.

▸ Microbiota plays a crucial role overseeing the body's two immune systems (innate and adaptive), helping them learn how to identify pathogens and managing levels of inflammation.

## intestinal barrier function

A healthy microbiota supports the maintenance of the gastrointestinal tract's integrity. A strong intestinal wall prevents a common condition called increased intestinal permeability ('leaky gut'). This inflammatory condition allows larger molecules and pathogens to escape through an ineffective intestinal wall into the bloodstream.

*Gather round for one of my favourite anti-inflammatory, intestinal-healing drinks: add a teaspoon of coconut oil to turmeric latte and let it cool a little before adding a teaspoon of L-glutamine powder.*

*Probiotic supplements are living beneficial bacteria, so no hot drinks or hot food at least 20 minutes before or after taking them or they will burn. Ouch.*

# food reactions

Experiencing unwanted symptoms after eating, from digestive issues, nausea, bloating and diarrhoea, to joint pain, sneezing and rashes, are not uncommon. However, it's very important to find out whether the body is experiencing an allergy, sensitivity or intolerance, as it could be the difference between discomfort or something that is potentially life-threatening. The good news is the body's immune system and intestinal microbiota continually evolves, meaning some of these reactions may disappear over time. Clever and brilliant microbiota.

## ALLERGIES

The body can develop an allergy at any age and to any food. Studies have suggested that eight foods – milk, eggs, fish, shellfish, peanuts and other nuts, wheat and soya beans – are responsible for 90 per cent of allergic reactions, and that approximately 1–2 per cent of the UK population has genuine food allergies. An allergic reaction is when the immune system reacts to something harmless with a completely overblown response, inducing symptoms that can range in severity from hives or rashes, abdominal pain, diarrhoea, vomiting and low blood pressure, to facial, lip, tongue or throat swelling, which leads to difficulty breathing. Some of these can be very dangerous and may progress into anaphylaxis, a life-threatening reaction where the entire body goes into shock in as little as a matter of minutes. *Allergies are extremely serious and anyone who experiences severe symptoms should contact a doctor or healthcare practitioner immediately.*

## FOOD SENSITIVITY

Sensitivities are generally considered to trigger an inflammatory immune response within the body, which creates additional symptoms. The irritated and inflamed intestinal wall allows partially digested food molecules to escape into the bloodstream, where they are mis-identified as pathogens and attacked.

These can cause uncomfortable symptoms that may be felt immediately, or even hours later, including abdominal pain, anxiety, bloating, brain fog, diarrhoea, fatigue, headaches, heartburn, joint pain, nausea and rashes.

Sensitivities have been linked to autoimmune conditions such as multiple sclerosis (MS), lupus, rheumatoid arthritis and psoriasis.

One of the main culprits for causing a food sensitivity is probably gluten, and annoyingly a sensitivity to gluten increases the chances of finding other proteins like dairy, eggs and grains problematic, too. Gluten does not like to party alone. Other common sensitivities include corn, soy, yeast, nightshades (tomatoes, aubergines, peppers), nuts (peanuts, walnuts, cashews, almonds), lentils and chickpeas.

## FOOD INTOLERANCE

Food intolerances are what most people experience. More often than not, an intolerance is caused by digestive enzyme deficiencies or an inability to properly digest natural components in food. Symptoms include heartburn, bloating, flatulence, nausea, diarrhoea or constipation.

Triggers typically include sugars within certain vegetables (broccoli, garlic, onions), additives like MSG, the lactose in dairy, fermented foods (kimchi, tofu, kombucha, yogurt, tempeh), alcohol, shellfish, smoked meat, chocolate and caffeine. Fortunately, an intolerance may not be permanent. Foods can be cut out temporarily, before reintroducing them after six to eight weeks. See page 73 for how to do this safely.

# This is embarrassing . . . er, what is going on?

### ▶ Bloating and flatulence

Intolerances, low levels of digestive enzymes, an imbalanced microbiota, eating too quickly, artificial sweeteners, drinking carbonated drinks, gulping down air or not chewing properly are just some of the triggers. The large intestine's bacteria also produce gas when digesting fibres, starches and sugars that have not been absorbed in the small intestine. The intestinal lining will partially absorb the gas into the bloodstream to eventually be breathed out, while some will cause bloating. Soooo, high-fibre diets can increase flatulence, but this is normal. And actually good for you.

### ▶ Constipation and diarrhoea

Constipation is typically the result of not including enough water and/or fibre in your diet. When the body is dehydrated, the large intestine absorbs too much water to help out, resulting in stools that are hard and difficult to pass. There are two types of fibre – digestible (soluble) and non-digestible (insoluble). While soluble fibre is important for regulating blood sugar levels, reducing cholesterol and balancing intestinal pH, insoluble fibre is the one that absorbs water, helping form easily passed stools and preventing constipation.

Diarrhoea is most frequently caused by a bacterial or viral infection, food intolerances and sensitivities or an imbalanced intestinal microbiota. The large intestine absorbs less water, to loosen stools and flush out the problem. This can cause the body to become dehydrated.

### ▶ Irritable Bowel Syndrome

Irritable Bowel Syndrome (IBS) affects the digestive tract and brings on symptoms such as bloating, flatulence, abdominal pain, constipation and diarrhoea. An imbalanced intestinal microbiota is thought to be one of the causes of IBS, triggering the immune system to generate an inflammatory response.

### ▶ Indigestion

Indigestion is the result of stomach acid being pushed up towards the unprotected lining of oesophagus, causing a burning sensation and symptoms like heartburn, nausea and burping. This can be triggered in many different ways, including eating too much or too late at night, smoking, stress and being overweight, as well as fried, fatty or spicy foods, alcohol, coffee, fizzy drinks, chocolate, peppermint, tomatoes and citrus fruit.

BUT... be careful. These symptoms can also be caused by low stomach acid, which is much more common than most people think, so taking antacids will only inhibit what little stomach acid is being produced in the first place, ultimately making the problem worse. Low levels of gastric acid can allow orally ingested pathogens to flourish, causing infections and gastrointestinal damage, as well as significantly suppressing the absorption of vitamins and minerals.

# So what do we do?

## the four 'R' protocol

The Four R Protocol approach – Remove, Replace, Reinoculate and Repair – is a highly effective method commonly used to investigate and address different digestive symptoms, as well as headaches, problematic skin, turbulent hormones, erratic moods and a weakened immune system.

## 1 remove
**Start by identifying potential triggers and try to remove them.**

### PROBLEMATIC FOODS
Begin with observation, removing the suspects from the diet for 2–3 weeks. Reintroduce them, one at a time, every 2–3 days, watching for any recurring symptoms. Gluten, dairy, eggs or grains are common triggers. For quicker answers, have a food intolerance or sensitivity blood test.

### STRESS
Stress is not just in the mind – it's a physical response where the hormone cortisol is released into the bloodstream. An excess of cortisol can create inflammation as well as impair the digestion and absorption process.

### PATHOGENS
One way to get rid of pathogens is by balancing the intestinal microbiota and increasing levels of beneficial bacteria. The third 'R' step (Reinoculate) explains how to do this. It's normal to have non-beneficial bacteria and yeasts, but when they start to overgrow, they compete with good bacteria for space. A more direct way to kill them off is by taking plant extracts with antimicrobial or antifungal properties:

▸ *Grapefruit seed extract, oregano oil, berberine, caprylic acid, uva ursi, manuka honey, garlic, goldenseal.*

### INFLAMMATORY FOODS
Certain types of food aggravate the intestinal lining. This varies from person to person, but try avoiding or minimising the following:

▸ *Processed meat (sausages, bacon, hot dogs).*
▸ *Refined carbohydrates and sugary foods (sweets, white bread, white rice, pasta, pastries, fizzy drinks, biscuits).*
▸ *Artificial trans fats (margarine, fried food).*
▸ *Excessive alcohol.*

**GP tip**
*The brain needs to think about food to start producing digestive enzymes. Always take a proper, focussed break when eating, chew properly and avoid all screens. Work, stress and food are not a good mix.*

*Three ways to help break down food naturally. 1/ Two tablespoons of apple cider vinegar in a little water at the onset of a rich meal to increase stomach acid. 2/ Bitter foods like rocket or chicory as a starter to stimulate enzyme production. 3/ Digestive enzymes containing papaya and pineapple for pudding.*

## 2 *replace*
### Address deficiencies and support digestion.

Low levels of digestive enzymes and stomach acid may result in partially digested food. These big particles will travel to the small intestine, where they will irritate the lining, causing sensitivities and intolerances, like an intestinal house of horrors. Fortunately, there are tricks to maintain healthy digestion and absorption.

### BITTER IS BETTER. SOUR IS POWER
The tongue has receptors that become activated by bitter foods, stimulating the salivary glands, stomach, liver and pancreas to produce digestive enzymes. There are more bitter receptors in the stomach, which tell the brain that enough food has been eaten. Strong bitter tastes include:
- *Rocket, chicory, radicchio, artichokes, dandelion greens.*

### WHEN IN DOUBT, SUPPLEMENT
Good-quality digestive enzyme supplements are an easy and convenient way to support digestion, particularly at the onset of a rich or protein-heavy meal. Similarly, there are lots of bitter tonics available, which I use in combination with supplements:
- *Supplements: should contain protease, lipase, amylase, pepsin and hydrochloric acid, which can be listed as betaine HCL.*
- *Bitter tonics: berberine, gentian, dandelion, burdock root, fennel seed or ginger. Add drops directly onto the tongue 5–10 minutes before eating, or as directed.*

*Add aromatic bitters to cocktails and then raise a toast to the genius who discovered this would help digestion.*

## 3 *reinoculate*
### Increase good bacteria to help restore a healthy, balanced microbiota.

### PREBIOTICS
Prebiotics are the non-digestible plant fibres that feed and promote the growth of probiotic bacteria (the kind we love and want). They are mostly found in fruit, vegetables, beans and pulses.

- *Leeks, onions, asparagus, bananas, garlic, Jerusalem artichokes, dandelion greens, agave, wheat bran, apples, strawberries, nuts (almonds, cashews, walnuts), seeds (pumpkin, hemp, chia, flax), psyllium, oats, celery, beans, lentils, peas.*

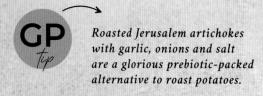

*Roasted Jerusalem artichokes with garlic, onions and salt are a glorious prebiotic-packed alternative to roast potatoes.*

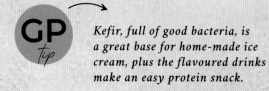

*Kefir, full of good bacteria, is a great base for home-made ice cream, plus the flavoured drinks make an easy protein snack.*

## PROBIOTICS

Naturally fermented foods are widely available to buy and all the rage right now, thanks to their ability to help maintain a balanced intestinal microbiota. The fermentation process produces the live microorganisms that help break down nutrients and increase absorption:

▸ *Sauerkraut, kimchi, miso, tempeh, probiotic (live) yogurt, kefir, kombucha.*

## SUPPLEMENT SUPERSTARS

Probiotic supplements can supply the digestive tract with a healthy mixture of beneficial bacteria. They are different to fermented foods in that probiotic supplements stay in the digestive tract and can colonise there.

The potency is measured in colony-forming units (CFU), so the general rule of thumb is the higher the dose (up to anything like 450 billion), the better the results. It's hard to overdo probiotics (some people may experience bloating, but it's rare), so the only real consideration is that as the CFU increases, so does the price. I would recommend taking probiotics for a month at least and then every other month if needed:

▸ *Digestive issues and imbalances: a multi-strain probiotic with a minimum of 30–50 billion CFU.*
▸ *Immune support and maintenance of everyday health: a multi-strain probiotic containing a minimum of 10 billion CFU.*

**GP** *tip*

*Miso paste is incredibly versatile – use it in dressings and soups or as a glaze for white fish.*

**GP** *tip*

*Organic home-made bone broth, rich in minerals, collagen and protein, helps heal and support the intestinal lining.*

## 4 repair

Create a healthy environment that encourages the digestive tract to heal.

## ANTI-INFLAMMATORY FOODS

▸ **L-glutamine foods:** *chicken, fish, cabbage, spinach, dairy, tofu, lentils, beans.*
▸ **Spices:** *turmeric, ginger, pepper, cinnamon.*
▸ **Phytonutrient-rich foods:** *kale, raspberries, peppers, blackberries, pumpkins.*
▸ **Omega-3:** *oily fish (salmon, mackerel, sardines), nuts (walnuts, almonds, cashews), seeds (pumpkin, flax, chia).*

## INTESTINAL HEALING

Introduce these supplements 2–3 weeks after starting to take probiotics.

▸ *Multi-nutrient that includes zinc and vitamins A, D and E.*
▸ *For faster results, add L-glutamine, L-glycine, omega-3, deglycyrrhizinated licorice, slippery elm, aloe vera, curcumin.*

### Superhero supplements

- Anti-microbials – grapefruit seed extract, oregano, berberine
- L-glutamine
- Wheatgrass
- Digestive enzyme complex (including HCL)
- Probiotics
- Slippery elm
- Curcumin

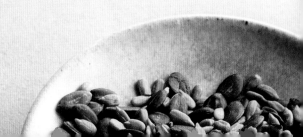

# 6/

# hair,
# skin,
# nails

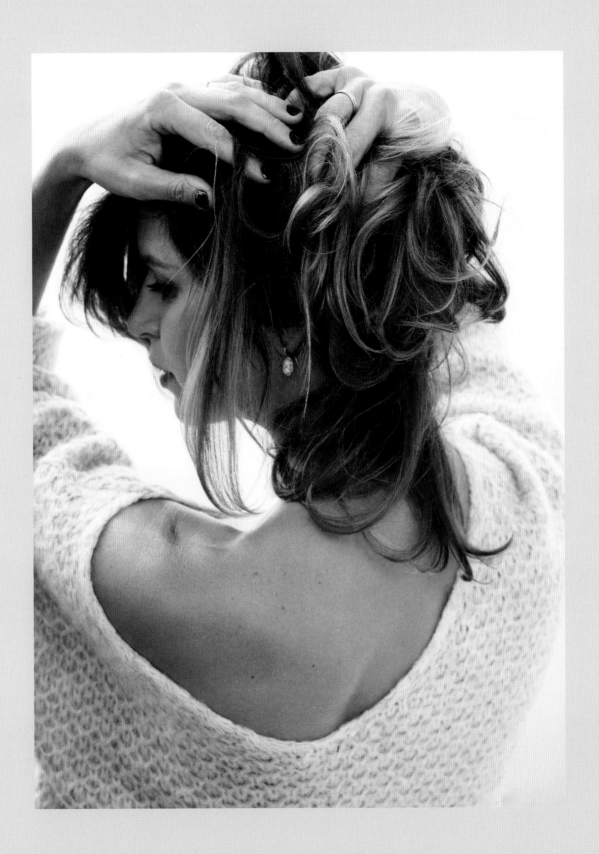

*do you ...*

- ☐ have dry, flaky skin?
- ☐ experience skin blemishes?
- ☐ have brittle or weak nails?
- ☐ sunbathe regularly?
- ☐ have lacklustre hair?

Our hair, skin and nails are an important aspect of our external appearance, but can also be a reflection of what may be going on inside our bodies. With so many jobs and systems to control, the body has to prioritise what contributes to our survival, often leaving them at the back of the queue. However, they play a valuable role in keeping us dry, warm and dextrous.

# skin

The body's largest organ, skin is flexible, waterproof and insulating. It acts as a barrier against pathogens and toxins and assists in our sensory experience of the world.

## what does the skin do?

- ▶ **Protection**
  It protects us against bacteria, cold, heat and many other external factors.
- ▶ **Sensation**
  Nerve endings in the skin help the body to identify temperature, pressure, pain and pleasure.
- ▶ **Strength and flexibility**
  Collagen fibres give skin its strength, while elastin allows it to stretch, giving freedom and flexibility to move.

- ▶ **Temperature regulation**
  The body manages thermoregulation through the skin, by making hairs stand on end to keep us warm or producing sweat to reduce heat.
- ▶ **Storage**
  Skin stores water and lipids.
- ▶ **Vitamin D production**
  Vitamin D is synthesised through the skin when it is exposed to the sun's UV rays.

# how is skin structured?

Skin is composed of three layers. The top, visible layer is the epidermis, a waterproof barrier made of keratin. The dermis in the middle is the thickest, formed by a web of structural proteins containing collagen and elastin. Elastin allows the skin to return to 'normal' after it is pinched or stretched, while collagen gives strength and structural support. The deepest layer is the hypodermis, which is composed mainly of subcutaneous fat and keeps the skin cushioned.

# what will affect the skin?

## AGEING

As the body ages, its systems ease their pace. While the skin continues to lose dead cells, the rate at which it generates new ones slows, as does its delivery of nutrients, water and blood flow, resulting in less-nourished skin. Reduced collagen levels behave a bit like a ladder with rungs removed – the fibres become shorter and thinner, with the dermis less filled and plumped. This weaker structure can lead to collapse, causing wrinkles. Collagen production decreases by approximately 1 per cent a year from the age of 20, with the skin becoming less robust to environmental stressors, smoking, UV rays and oxidative stress.

The good news (finally!) is that encouraging blood flow and lymphatic drainage to reduce toxins and fluid build-up, as well as supplying the skin with plenty of nutrients, can also support the production of collagen and elastin.

## INFLAMMATORY SKIN CONDITIONS

▸ **Eczema** – another very common complaint with symptoms that can include dry, inflamed, itchy skin and sometimes blisters. It has been linked to anything from fragrances, soaps, pollen, stress and foods that include nuts and dairy.

▸ **Acne** – a very common condition linked to hormone imbalances, as well as some nutrient deficiencies. It triggers excess sebum (oil) production, which allows bacteria to develop and cause breakouts.

▸ **Rosacea** – inflammation of the skin's blood vessels and sebaceous (oil) glands can result in flushed complexions, redness and blemishes. The exact cause is unclear, but low stomach acid, imbalanced intestinal microflora and dietary triggers like dairy, caffeine, alcohol and spice are all implicated.

▸ **Psoriasis** – presenting as red, itchy and scaly patches, it is typically found on knees, elbows, the scalp and the torso. It is an autoimmune condition linked to nutrient deficiencies that has cycles of flare-ups and remission.

## SUN EXPOSURE

When skin is exposed to the sun, it increases production of the pigment melanin to prevent burning and UV rays penetrating its deeper layers – causing skin to tan. This change in colour fades as these darker cells approach the surface, where they then flake off to be replaced by new ones. Over time, sun exposure can lead to a reduction in elasticity and increase ageing, as skin cells become damaged or destroyed.

GP *tip*
*To increase their absorption, take collagen supplements in hydrolysed form (also known as collagen peptides).*

GP *tip*
*A good-quality anti-inflammatory nutrient combination will cut down the number of supplements you take on a daily basis.*

# hair

The body has 5 million hairs all over it, which grow on a rotation over the course of our lives. Each scalp follicle typically grows a hair for 2–5 years, after which it falls out and is replaced in a cycle that is repeated 20–25 times in a lifetime.

Much like skin, hair colour is determined by the amount of melanin pigment present in it; the more there is, the darker the hair. Red hair is specifically created by a pigment called pheomelanin. Genetics determine our natural hair colour, while hormones and environmental changes also play a role in any changes that occur, like fair-haired children becoming darker with age.

## what does hair do?

> **Protection**
> Hair on the head protects the scalp from the sun. Nostril hair filters any inhaled particles, preventing them from getting into the respiratory system. Eyelashes help to stop debris getting into the eyes.

> **Regulation of body temperature**
> Hair traps heat, but also helps the evaporation of sweat, allowing the body to cool down.

> **Sensory reception**
> Hair roots detect touch, sending signals to the brain which it translates into sensation.

 *As little as 70g (2½oz) of kale, the hair and skin superfood, will exceed your daily recommended intake of vitamin C. It's also rich in iron and beta-carotene. Top marks all round.*

## hair structure

The hair is formed in two parts – the follicle, which lives under the skin, and the shaft, which is the keratin structure above the skin and is the part we can see. As the follicle bulb, it needs a constant supply of oxygen and nutrients. This enables its cells to divide quickly – as fast as every day or two – resulting in its growth. Amazing, or annoying, for those of us who have to have our roots done.

 *Have half a grapefruit with breakfast every morning for springy, vitamin C-infused skin and hair.*

 *Zinc and iron supplements are essential for hair and nails, but compete for absorption, so don't take them at the same time.*

# what can scare the hair?

Heated implements, damaging products and dying it neon pink can all upset the hair, but it is also strongly affected by diet. As the body does not deem hair to be a vital organ (it needs to watch *Fleabag*: 'HAIR IS EVERYTHING') its nutritional needs are not prioritised. That is why imbalances or deficiencies of nutrients such as vitamin D or B vitamins can commonly trigger hair loss.

### HORMONES

Hair loves oestrogen, which is why its levels will impact hair growth and loss. It's common for women to experience a surge of hair growth during pregnancy that accompanies a rise in oestrogen. When these levels drop after the pregnancy, the cycle resets itself and this extra hair very often falls out. This can be alarming, but it is normal. A reduction in hair volume is also common during menopause, when oestrogen levels naturally begin to decrease.

The thyroid, which is responsible for the speed at which things happen in the body, can impact hair. An underactive thyroid can lead to a decrease in oestrogen production, with hair taking a hit. Premature baldness, which tends to affect women to a lesser extent, is caused by a genetic predisposition and increased levels of testosterone.

 *Don't throw fish skin away – it's even higher in collagen and omega-3 than the fish itself, so eat it fried and crispy.*

 *Boil a couple of eggs in the morning and put them in the fridge for a hair-loving, vitamin B, protein-rich snack.*

# nails

Like the hair, nails are made of keratin, but are stronger and harder. Their primary role is to provide protection, strength, gripping and sensation, as well as increase our ability to perform detailed tasks (like threading a needle).

Fingernails have a higher blood supply compared to toenails, as they are closer to the heart, which is why they grow faster. However, both are reliant on a steady supply of nutrients to maintain their health, flexibility and appearance. Nails can provide a useful indication into the rate of circulation to the extremities, as well as signs of imbalances within the body.

> ▸ **Brittle, soft or weak nails** can suggest an overworked liver or a deficiency in calcium, iron, zinc or B vitamins (biotin).
>
> ▸ **White spots** may be a harmless indication of past nail trauma or a sign of zinc or calcium deficiency.
>
> ▸ **Grooves or ridges** in the nails are a normal sign of ageing, but also may be due to a lack of vitamin B12, vitamin A or protein intake.
>
> ▸ **Flat or concave nails** can be a symptom of iron-deficiency anaemia, or (less commonly) liver conditions or an underactive thyroid.

# So what do we do?

The best way to support the skin's integrity, particularly as it begins to age, is through consuming nutrients that encourage collagen production, foods that contain collagen and anti-inflammatory nutrients. When it comes to hair, it's all about nourishing the follicle with targeted nutrients and balanced hormone levels (see the Hormones chapter on page 84), which also support nail growth to keep them strong and healthy.

## COLLAGEN – the nutrient king

As collagen is a protein, the body will have to break it down into amino acids because it cannot be absorbed whole. These amino acids will then be reconstructed and used as building blocks – but they may or may not be directed to collagen production, potentially being used for other jobs like repairing a sore ankle. This is why it's important to include nutrients that support its production, not just collagen itself.

## COLLAGEN HERO – vitamin C

This nutrient has a major role in collagen synthesis. It offers antioxidant support and prevents free radical damage caused by UV exposure. Similarly, it helps protect nails and hair:

▶ *Fruit (kiwis, raspberries, blueberries, citrus, pineapple, mango), vegetables (sprouts, cauliflower, cabbage, kale, peppers, chard).*

## COLLAGEN SUPERFOODS

These foods can amplify the body's production levels, as well as delivering collagen itself to keep skin, hair and nails healthy and strong.

▶ **Fish** – *especially oily fish, is one of the best food sources of collagen. Its protein content and high levels of omega-3 fatty acids also increase the strength of hair follicles and keep nails healthy, supple and shiny.*

▶ **Eggs** – *a double whammy of collagen content and collagen-producing amino acids, as well as hyaluronic acid, which is fantastic for plumping the skin by attracting water. The yolk is also high in B vitamins and choline, which are essential for hair growth.*

▶ **Bone broth** – *animal bones contain collagen and other amino acids responsible for its production, which, along with many additional nutrients, makes this a superfood.*

*Make home-made bone broth with 2kg (4½lbs) of organic bones in a large pot filled with water. Add a dash of apple cider vinegar, your favourite vegetables and spices and simmer on a low heat for 12 hours. I like it as a nightcap.*

*A home-made face mask of avocado, honey and live yogurt blends nourishing good fats, anti-inflammatory properties and beneficial bacteria to make your skin bouncier than a trampoline.*

## MAGIC MINERALS
### Zinc and copper

Zinc is essential for producing and maintaining collagen and keratin, as well as being one of the best minerals for acne and breakouts, as it reduces excessive oil production in the skin and can protect against inflammation. It also strengthens brittle or weak hair and nails (which can be a sign of a zinc deficiency) and supports growth. Copper supports collagen function, repairing it if it becomes damaged to make sure it stays strong and healthy.

▸ *Zinc and copper are both found in seafood (oysters, crab, clams), seeds (pumpkin, sunflower, sesame, chia, flax, hemp), nuts (almonds, cashews, walnuts, Brazil nuts, hazelnuts), tofu, lentils, mushrooms (shiitake, button, portobello).*

## SPIRULINA – the star from the sea

The marine algae spirulina is rich in nutrients and protein, which provide the amino acid building blocks that are used to make collagen. It's also a fantastic non-animal-derived protein powerhouse that supports hair, skin and nails.

## ANTI-INFLAMMATORY NUTRIENTS

Inflammatory skin conditions like acne, rosacea, eczema and psoriasis will all benefit from anti-inflammatory nutrients. They are highly beneficial in supporting the skin against premature ageing and dry skin conditions. Vitamin D and omega-3 are also beneficial for brittle nails and helping create new hair follicles:

▸ *Omega-3 – oily fish (salmon, mackerel, sardines, trout, tuna), nuts (almonds, Brazil nuts, walnuts, hazelnuts, cashews), seeds (pumpkin, sunflower, chia, flax, hemp).*
▸ *Vitamin D – oily fish (mackerel, salmon, sardines, herring), red meat (beef, pork, lamb), liver, mushrooms (chestnut, shiitake, portobello, button), egg yolks and whole milk, careful sun exposure.*
▸ *Curcumin – found in turmeric.*

**GP** *Tip*

*Make spirulina energy balls with 225g (8oz) pitted dates, 2 teaspoons of melted coconut oil, 2 tablespoons of pumpkin seeds and 1 tablespoon of spirulina. Blitz everything in a blender, form the mixture into 4 balls and refrigerate.*

## VITAMIN B COMPLEXION

B vitamins are involved in multiple processes, including quick skin cell regeneration, which prevents dry and flaky skin, plus biotin (vitamin B7) plays a crucial role in the synthesis of hair and nails. All B vitamins are water-soluble, which means the body cannot hold onto them for long – that's why it's essential to make sure they are regularly consumed:

▸ *Eggs, dairy (cheese, milk, natural live yogurt), fish (salmon, tuna, mackerel), shellfish (oysters, clams), dark leafy vegetables (kale, spinach, cavolo nero), wholegrains (brown rice, quinoa, rye), beans, chickpeas, meat (beef, pork, chicken, turkey, liver, kidney).*

*Superhero supplements*

- Collagen peptides
- Vitamin C
- Zinc
- Hyaluronic acid
- Vitamin B complex
- Omega-3
- Red/purple/blue superfood powders

# 7/

# hormone harmony

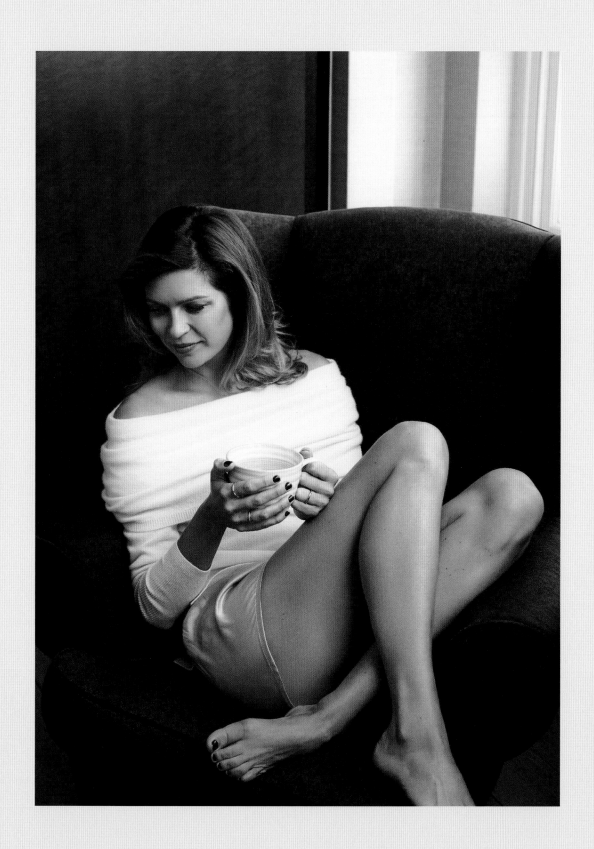

*do you* ...

- ☐ feel wired and stressed on a regular basis?
- ☐ regularly crave sugar?
- ☐ find PMS or menopause symptoms challenging?
- ☐ notice that recently you've gained weight and have less energy?
- ☐ often feel tired and moody?

Hormones are the body's chemical messengers and are produced by a number of glands, which are collectively known as the endocrine system. They travel around the bloodstream to targeted organs, tissues and cells, delivering information through special receptors on the recipient cell's membrane.

There are 50 types of hormones and they play a number of important roles in different areas around the body. If we went into detail on all of them, this chapter would be longer than *The Decline and Fall of the Roman Empire*. Instead, I'm going to focus on the hormones that I see issues with most commonly in my patients. Hormones are so interlinked that if one area is playing up, it will almost inevitably affect the others.

# adrenal hormones

The adrenal glands, which live above the kidneys, secrete a number of steroid hormones that help regulate the metabolism, blood pressure and immune system, as well as the stress hormones adrenaline and cortisol.

## 1 ADRENALINE AND NORADRENALINE

These stress hormones trigger an immediate response from the body to a perceived threat, known as 'fight or flight'. The brain's hypothalamus will immediately sound the alarm, unleashing a flurry of signals that tell the adrenal glands to rush out stress hormones, including adrenaline. This surge increases the heart rate and contractility, blood flow, oxygen and energy levels, putting the body on high alert.

## 2 CORTISOL

Most of the body's cells have cortisol receptors, which means that its role extends beyond that as a stress hormone. It is involved with regulating the circadian rhythm, metabolism, blood pressure and blood sugar levels, supporting memory function and suppressing inflammation. It also helps balance the body's salt and water levels.

# the acute stress response

The body experiences 2 types of stress response: acute and chronic. When acute, the brain and body experience a quick-fire sequence of events that prepare it for the sudden burst of energy it might need for fight or flight.

- ▸ The brain identifies the threat, triggering the hypothalamus to immediately green-light the body's stress response.

- ▸ Adrenaline and noradrenaline are released into the bloodstream.

- ▸ Breathing rate, heart rate and blood pressure all increase.

- ▸ Blood flow is diverted from less crucial mechanisms like digestion (hence why no one feels like eating during acute stress) and sent instead to the muscles, heart and lungs.

- ▸ The body is ready to run from the lion/ unscheduled Zoom meeting/scary cat next door.

When this period of hypervigilance has subsided, the body can then settle again as it breaks down the adrenaline and noradrenaline it no longer needs, removing them from circulation. However, the hypothalamus cues round two of its response with a new wave of stress hormones.

Typically after about 15 minutes, the adrenal glands secrete cortisol into the bloodstream, where it releases stored glucose. This will energise the muscles and prepare the brain to issue instructions for tissue repair, if needed. Cortisol will also trigger the liver to continue to suppress non-crucial systems like digestion and subdue inflammation. The body and brain are therefore kept in a state of alert, with energy at the ready, should it be needed. When this is over, the body once again works to break down the cortisol it no longer needs and to remove it from the bloodstream. We can now sit down, have a stiff drink and recover.

*If it's too early in the day for a G&T, try the other kind – green tea. It contains L-theanine, a naturally calming amino acid, which will help lower the effects of cortisol raging around the body.*

*Stress-reducing adaptogenic herbs work wonders, especially when combined. They all have different benefits and will work happily alongside each other.*

# *The chronic stress response*

It's important to remember that we need to be able to experience stress and that it's completely normal. The problem is that we are now experiencing it much too regularly, thanks to the pressures of modern life – too much worrying, too many deadlines, constantly pinging phones. While these stresses are not life-threatening, they're ongoing, which means the body continues to respond to them by persistently releasing cortisol, leaving it constantly wired. This is chronic stress, which is not natural or normal for the body and undermines the effectiveness of stress hormones when they are actually needed. The consequences of cortisol can be varied:

### ▸ Digestive problems
Stress can play havoc with digestion, as cortisol redirects blood meant for the brain, stomach and intestine to the muscles. This disruption can result in mean digestive issues, such as irritable bowel syndrome (IBS), constipation, diarrhoea and indigestion.

### ▸ Weight gain
Cortisol contributes to the storage of unused nutrients in adipose tissue and stimulates the appetite in order to increase energy needed to deal with the potential 'threat'.

### ▸ Mental health issues
High levels of cortisol can suppress the production of serotonin, causing mood swings, irritability and depression. It can also trigger or exacerbate anxiety.

### ▸ Disturbed sleep
Cortisol plays an important role in the circadian rhythm, helping to wake the body up in the morning. Too much cortisol can interfere with the sleep cycle, resulting in exhaustion and moodiness during the day.

### ▸ Cardiovascular disruption
Persistent surges in stress hormones have the potential to increase blood pressure, which can damage arteries and blood vessels, and therefore increase the risk of cardiovascular diseases.

## *the cortisol kidnapper*

Cortisol is a formidable old-school diva, expecting everyone and everything to succumb to its demands. The body tends to prioritise adrenal hormone production because it is more integral to survival. That's why a constant supply of cortisol in the bloodstream will inevitably start competing with the production of other hormones. Hormone imbalances of all kinds will inevitably follow. Excess cortisol can also suppress and slow the production of thyroid hormones, leading to insulin resistance and imbalanced blood sugar levels.

# reproductive hormones

Reproductive hormones are central to the body's sexual development and reproductive function, as well as being involved in bone, muscle and hair growth, and the regulation of cholesterol, inflammation and fat distribution. Female reproductive hormones are predominantly made in the ovaries, and men's are mostly produced in the testes. While men do produce progesterone and oestrogen, and women produce testosterone, we will be focusing on the dominant levels of progesterone and oestrogen in females and testosterone in males.

## TESTOSTERONE
Essential for sexual development, testosterone is a critical player in the male reproductive hormone squad. It helps with the production of sperm and red blood cells, and regulates libido, metabolic function, muscle and bone mass, fat distribution and cognitive function.

## OESTROGEN AND PROGESTERONE
These are part of the female reproductive hormone team managing the menstrual cycle, fertility, pregnancy and sexual development.

Oestrogen builds up the lining of the uterus wall during the first half of the cycle, and triggers menstruation if the egg is unfertilised. If conception occurs, they work together to develop the pregnancy. Oestrogen is also key for bone development, cardiovascular health, how energy is expended and the regulation of appetite. Progesterone is the on-site uterus-lining manager. Its levels drop in response to an unfertilised egg, triggering menstruation, but rise in response to conception to help the development of the foetus.

# PMS and the menopause

## PREMENSTRUAL SYNDROME (PMS)
Around 80 per cent of women experience a range of emotional and physical symptoms including cramping, irritability, breast tenderness, bloating and low energy. These can last from one day to two weeks before a woman gets her period and they usually subside shortly after menstruation has begun. PMS is actually caused by an imbalance between oestrogen and progesterone. If there is too much oestrogen or too little progesterone, this can cause what is known as oestrogen dominance – and that is what exacerbates the symptoms of PMS. While PMS symptoms vary, most are perfectly normal, within reason. However, wanting to smash the place up in a wild rage on a monthly basis is not something that has to be shrugged off as 'that's just the way it is'. Lifestyle and dietary changes can have a huge impact on symptoms.

## MENOPAUSE
Menopause is the result of the natural decline of reproductive hormone production. As with PMS, symptoms differ – some women go through it with very little trouble, while others may experience anything from hot flushes and fluctuating moods, to insomnia and night sweats. Nutritional intervention and lifestyle changes during menopause can be incredibly beneficial. Excess weight has been shown to increase the severity of symptoms, so for those who need to, shedding a few pounds may significantly improve the experience.

# thyroid hormones

The thyroid gland, which sits along the larynx, is shaped like a butterfly with two lobes. Its two hormones, thyroxine (T4) and triiodothyronine (T3), play a major role in the body's metabolic rate, heart health, digestive and cognitive function, muscle and bone growth and development. Thyroid hormones are the body's speed moderators, making sure everything is running at the rate it should. For example, if the heart pumps too slowly, the brain will send a message to the thyroid telling it to release hormones to get a message to the heart that it needs to pick up the pace.

If the body's temperature drops too low or if concentration seems to be flagging, it is the thyroid that will make sure everything is brought back up to the appropriate speed. It can also help the body lose weight by increasing the basal metabolic rate, which is responsible for the amount of energy needed when the body is resting. The thyroid signals to the cells throughout the body to work harder, firing up the metabolism.

## hypothyroidism

Hypothyroidism is a relatively common condition that occurs when the thyroid gland is not able to produce enough hormones. When this happens, the body may experience a kind of functional 'slow down', the effects of which may start out as mild and only develop gradually as the hormone levels begin to drop. Symptoms can include changes in mood, fatigue, feeling cold, dry skin, constipation and, most obviously, an increase in weight. Common causes of a slow thyroid can be iodine deficiency and high levels of cortisol due to chronic stress.

## appetite hormones

**LEPTIN**
Known as the satiety hormone, leptin is mostly secreted in fat cells, but also in the stomach, heart and muscle. Its job is to balance energy and manage appetite levels, making it important for reducing overall body fat and weight as it regulates long-term food intake.

**GHRELIN**
The hunger hormone ghrelin is mostly secreted by the stomach lining and stimulates the appetite when the body needs more energy. Its levels are at their highest just before a meal, lowering when it has finished.

## leptin resistance

As leptin is produced by fat cells, its levels are proportionate to the amount of fat on the body. More fat means more leptin – which should result in reducing food intake, as it's leptin's job to tell the brain enough has been eaten. The irony is, excess weight can cloud the brain's sensitivity to these increased levels. Instead of understanding that it is full, the body continues to feel hungry, worrying it doesn't have enough fat stored, resulting in weight gain. This is leptin resistance.

# So what do we do?

It is essential to look after the endocrine system as a whole, as all hormones are made of similar nutirents and respond to the same lifestyle changes. An imbalance in one will often mean an imbalance in others, so while there are a few specific recommendations, my advice is to take care of the house, not just one room in it.

## HORMONES + FRIENDLY BACTERIA

Who knew (obviously I did) that our intestinal microbiota and hormones have a very intimate relationship? The intestinal microbiota not only produces hormones, it also signals to the endocrine glands with instructions on the amount of hormones they should be making and when they should be released. Reason number 958 why a healthy, balanced diet is so important. Fermented foods increase the number of healthy bacteria in the intestine:

▸ *Kefir, natural live yogurt, kombucha, tempeh, miso, sauerkraut, kimchi.*

## GOOD SLEEP = HAPPY HORMONES

Hormones love a good night's sleep. Of course they do. Good-quality sleep helps to keep stress and hunger hormones in check, while poor sleep leaves hormones confused and erratic, disrupting cortisol levels throughout the day. As John Lennon once said, 'Give sleep a chance.'

▸ *Be mindful of bedtime habits – no screens, keep the bedroom temperature on the cooler side, jot down any badgering thoughts and try to go to bed/get up at a similar time.*

▸ *Balance blood sugar levels throughout the day to avoid spikes or lows around bedtime. Eat regularly and make sure protein is included in every meal or snack.*

## ESSENTIAL FATTY ACIDS (EFAs)

EFAs form part of the building blocks that make hormones as well as allowing them to signal their messages across the body effectively. The body is unable to produce essential fatty acids, so they need to be included as part of a balanced diet. Omega-3 is a highly effective anti-inflammatory, so it's especially beneficial because inflammation can be a common side effect of hormonal imbalances. It has been shown to benefit the more challenging symptoms of menopause, insufficient thyroid function and overworked adrenals. The moral of the story being: omega-3 fatty acids are extremely important for hormones. I would throw a fish at you if I had to, to get this point across – or omega-3 supplements if no fish were available:

▸ *Oily fish (salmon, herring, mackerel, sardines, tuna), or vegetarian sources like nuts (walnuts, almonds, hazelnuts), seeds (flax, chia, sunflower, hemp, pumpkin).*

**GP**
*Tip*

*Smoked salmon and scrambled eggs is an omega-3 breakfast of epic proportions. Add half an avocado to further boost the good fat content and your hormones will want to throw a party for you.*

## ADOPTING ADAPTOGENS

Adaptogens are plants that have been used for centuries in traditional medicine, naturally encouraging the body to cope with the effects of stress, as well as helping build resistance to it. They also play a role regulating hormones by assisting in the balance of blood sugar and insulin, improving the mood and supporting thyroid and adrenal function:

► *Ashwagandha, Siberian ginseng, rhodiola, schisandra, licorice, maca, holy basil.*

## MAX OUT ON MAGNESIUM

Magnesium is nature's relaxant, helping the body to wind down. There is nothing this amazing nutrient is not good for when it comes to hormones. As well as being involved with the general production of both thyroid and reproductive hormones, magnesium helps to keep oestrogen and progesterone balanced and is especially good at easing muscle tension and PMS cramps. During periods of stress and anxiety, the body uses up more magnesium, making it even more important to increase the intake of this miraculous mineral. Plus, having plenty in the body's system helps to control excess production of cortisol.

► *Magnesium levels are hard to increase through diet alone, but supplements are amazing, and often come combined with adaptogens and B vitamins.*

► *Soak in a warm bath of magnesium flakes (magnesium chloride) for at least 20 minutes to destress.*

► *Magnesium-rich foods – dark green leafy vegetables (spinach, kale, cavolo nero, collard greens, Swiss chard), seeds (pumpkin, hemp, flax, sesame, chia), nuts (almonds, cashews, peanuts), beans, chickpeas, lentils, grains (quinoa, brown rice, buckwheat), dark chocolate (65–70 per cent cocoa – watch caffeine content).*

*Take adaptogen supplements or add them in powder form to smoothies, porridge, cereal, home-made energy bars and lattes.*

*Magnesium glycinate is a fantastic supplement, as the addition of the amino acid glycine has a soothing effect on the brain, plus this combination is very easy for the body to absorb. Dream team.*

## FANGIRLING OVER FIBRE

High-fibre diets are crucial in helping the body get rid of excess hormones, preventing their unwanted reabsorption. Fibre has the ability to bind to used hormones and carry them through the digestive tract:

► *Cruciferous vegetables (broccoli, Brussels sprouts, cabbage, kale), beans, pulses, wheat bran, oat bran, grains (quinoa, brown rice, rye), nuts, seeds, apples, pears, avocado.*

*When you're too busy to focus on your fibre intake, try a glucomannan or psyllium husk supplement, which can be taken as a capsule or powder. It's a natural soluble fibre that will help eliminate redundant hormones from the body.*

## TOO MUCH CAFFEINE = ANXIETY

I personally don't have anything against coffee and I'm unlikely to tell someone who loves it to cut it out completely. However, during periods of stress, caffeine will exacerbate the problem, because it over-stimulates the body when it is already overstimulated, triggering the adrenals to release more cortisol and reducing its ability to process the effects of stress. High levels of caffeine can lead to other stress-related symptoms like anxiety and insomnia, as well as compromise the de-stressing capabilities of magnesium and metabolism-boosting B vitamins within the body. Caffeine is found in:

▶   *Tea, coffee, soft drinks (particularly energy drinks) and cocoa beans (the higher the cocoa levels, the higher the caffeine).*

*If the thought of eliminating caffeine is traumatising, try green or white tea, which not only contains about half the amount found in black tea, but also has many other health benefits. Just try not to drink it on an empty stomach.*

## THE STRESSFUL SUGAR CYCLE

It's not uncommon to crave something sugary when feeling stressed or anxious. This is because sugar can suppress the hypothalamic-pituitary-adrenal axis in the brain that manages the body's response to stress. The body will believe it has found some relief from whatever is worrying it. However, this is short-lived, as the sugar spike will be followed by the inevitable dip, resulting in blood sugar imbalance and increased cortisol levels. The cravings will continue, the mood will worsen and the cycle will become increasingly harder to break.

*No one wants to be told to eat a handful of pumpkin seeds when they're angry (just leaving that here). If chocolate is non-negotiable (it does contain caffeine, which we want to avoid, but also de-stressing magnesium), then choose dark chocolate, which tends to be less sugary. And again, not on an empty stomach.*

## FRIENDS AND ENEMIES OF THE METABOLISM

Iodine is an absolutely essential mineral for the production of thyroid hormones. The highest sources of iodine come from the sea:

▶   *Fish and shellfish (cod, salmon, tuna, prawns), seaweed, eggs, dairy products.*

Goitrogens are compounds found in all kinds of healthy vegetables, but can prevent the absorption of iodine if regularly eaten raw:

▶   *Cruciferous vegetables (broccoli, cabbage, bok choy, kale, Brussels sprouts, cauliflower, collard greens), radishes, bamboo shoots, sweet potato, spinach.*

*The occasional bit of raw broccoli or coleslaw will not shut down the thyroid, so don't panic. Steaming these vegetables will reduce the negative effects of goitrogens by two-thirds, so be free to gorge on (lightly cooked) cabbage leaves as much as your heart desires.*

## PHYTOESTROGENS, THE MAGICAL BALANCERS

Derived from plants, these compounds are similar to oestrogen in structure, but have a milder effect. They bind to cell receptors before oestrogen gets the chance to. This is beneficial in two ways. The first is because it helps with oestrogen dominance, which is when too much oestrogen is produced or its production exceeds other reproductive hormones like progesterone. Symptoms include tender breasts, bloating, mood swings, headaches, weight gain, PMS, anxiety, hair loss, trouble sleeping, memory problems and fatigue.

Secondly, when the body is experiencing very low oestrogen levels, which typically happens during menopause, phytoestrogens can act as a gentle, natural hormone therapy, delivering a low level of oestrogen. They may not have as strong an effect as medication, but they come without any potential side effects:

▶ *Soy products (tofu, tempeh, miso), legumes (beans, lentils, chickpeas), seeds (flax, sesame), wholegrains (rye, oats, brown rice, buckwheat, millet, quinoa), alfalfa, mung beans, apples, sweet potatoes, carrots, liquorice root, red clover.*

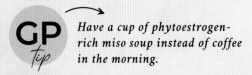

*Have a cup of phytoestrogen-rich miso soup instead of coffee in the morning.*

*Wash new clothes before wearing them to reduce contact with endocrine-disrupting chemicals that are commonly found on them.*

## EXCESS WEIGHT

As leptin gets produced in fat cells, losing weight will decrease its levels in the body, helping to break the vicious cycle of leptin resistance. Excess oestrogen that is also made by fat cells is linked to many chronic conditions, so losing weight will help to rebalance it and therefore all the reproductive hormones. Weight loss has also been shown to reduce insulin resistance, preventing chronic inflammation associated with higher levels of body fat.

## ENDOCRINE DISRUPTORS

Endocrine-disrupting chemicals (EDCs) are found in everything. They can mimic or interfere with hormone production and function, and are linked to immune, brain, reproductive and developmental imbalances.

Food, clothing, detergents, plastics, pesticides, fragrances, toys, the lining of metal food cans, skincare products, household cleaning products and pharmaceuticals are just a handful of places where EDCs will turn up. Don't lose your mind and think you have to leave your life and live in solitude under the sea in order to be safe. Everything is about balance and it's much better to think about how to reduce contact than ban them entirely.

▶ *Try shopping organic whenever possible, using stainless steel or ceramic cookware and swapping plastic for glass storage containers. Washing new clothes before wearing them and choosing clean personal and household products that are free from artificial fragrances will also help. See page 47.*

*My GP intermittent-fasting plans in the first chapter are the safest, easiest and most sustainable methods to shed excess pounds and balance hormone levels without starving or going mad.*

## TAKE A WALK ON THE MILD SIDE

Regular low-intensity exercise can really work wonders, even in small doses, as it's very effective at balancing hormones – with the added benefit of increased endorphins. Try riding a bike instead of taking a spin class or going for a brisk walk instead of a run to regulate hormone levels.

*I don't tend to recommend anything too cardio-heavy, like a manic HIIT class for those with overactive adrenals. Instead, mat classes such as Pilates or yoga, as clichéd as it might sound, are better options. The focus on breathing alone is a benefit in itself.*

## AND BREATHE… AAAAAAAHHHH

Being told how to breathe during stressful periods can seem a bit trite, but this is a good one. I love this breathing technique, because it's based on creating a physiological shift in the body when it is experiencing stress – and it does work. It's called the 4-7-8 technique. Breathing in for 4, holding for 7, breathing out for 8 overrules the sympathetic nervous system and triggers the parasympathetic nervous system to slow down the heart rate. It needs a few minutes to kick in, but it's worth putting the time in.

*Try the 4-7-8 breathing technique for 5–10 minutes (the longer the better) in the morning, after work, on the bus, in a boring meeting – anywhere – to reduce stress by physically calming the body.*

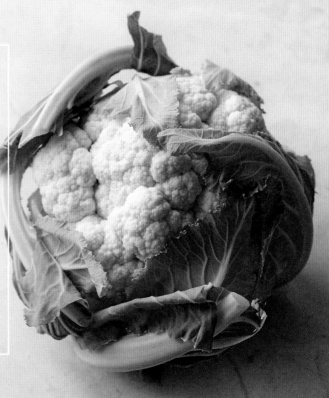

*Superhero supplements*

- Omega-3
- Probiotics
- Magnesium
- Vitamin B complex
- Glucomannan/psyllium fibre
- Vitamin D
- Adaptogens – ashwagandha, rhodiola, maca, reishi, moringa
- Black cohosh/ginseng/red clover – *menopause support*
- Selenium/iodine – *thyroid support*

# 8/

# healthy brain, happy mind

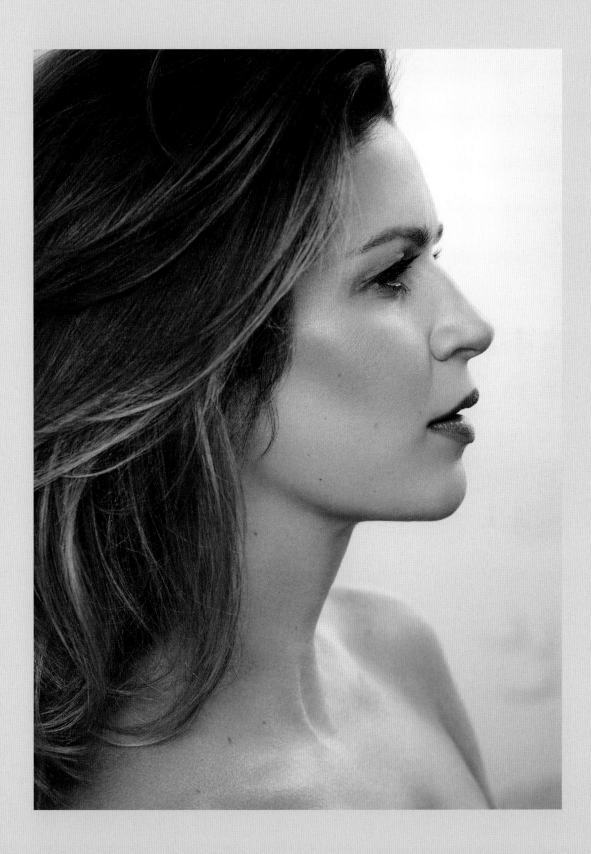

# the brilliant, baffling brain

The brain really is (irony) a mind-blowing organ which is believed to contain around 100 billion neurons, that make trillions of connections between them. It takes around 20 per cent of the body's calories to fuel this high-intensity engine room so that it can carry out its critical work. Brains are miraculous, adaptable, relentless, extraordinary – and, yes, greedy.

The brain forms one half of the central nervous system (the other half is the spinal cord) and in a nutshell, its job is to control the functions of the body and mind – everything from breathing, sleeping, eating and heart rate to thinking, learning, memory, reasoning, communication, attention, language and emotions. The simplest of tasks, like walking across a room or making a cup of tea, requires the brain to undertake thousands of different jobs, which most of us are completely oblivious to. We need this soft, grey, 1.4kg (3 pound) crown jewel to keep us healthy (and alive).

The brain is, of course, responsible for cognitive function. This refers to the mental processes that allow us to acquire, store, develop and retrieve information from the surrounding world and use this information to help navigate and understand our environment. We'll be focussing on how to balance moods and emotions, support memory and sharpen mental clarity. You might be an evil genius by the end (fingers crossed).

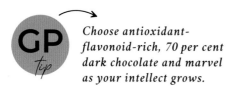

*Choose antioxidant-flavonoid-rich, 70 per cent dark chocolate and marvel as your intellect grows.*

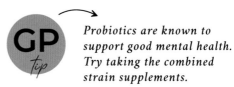

*Probiotics are known to support good mental health. Try taking the combined strain supplements.*

# emotions, feelings and moods

- **Emotions** are the quickest sensation to occur and the most intense. The brain responds to a trigger, immediately releasing chemicals throughout the body.

- **Feelings** are the brain and body's interpretation of emotions. The brain perceives the emotion and attaches meaning to it, resulting in a feeling. Feelings tend to last longer.

- **Moods** are the least acute and can usually be defined very generally as good or bad. Lasting longer than feelings, moods are not triggered by particular incidents and stimulate a less intense response. Weather, food, sleep, exercise and hormones can all influence mood.

Mental health is intricate, sensitive, unpredictable and often erratic, but what's important to remember is that it is not something that is just 'in the head', but a very real psychological experience that has myriad effects on the body. Human beings are capable of a wide, rich spectrum of emotions, and feeling low is one of them. However, if low moods linger for longer than a couple of weeks, or get worse, it could be a sign of depression, which is a clinical condition. It's really important to ask for help if this happens. Understanding the difference between a low mood and depression is vital, not only to help us recognise it in ourselves, but also in those around us.

# the limbic system

The limbic system is like the brain's control centre. The hippocampus is associated with learning, memory, spatial awareness and information storage, and the amygdala covers emotional identification, association and memory. The hypothalamus is responsible for the production and release of mood-associated chemicals.

# neurotransmitters

Each region of the limbic system releases neurotransmitters, which are chemical messengers that travel at speed to neurons (cells of the nervous system), muscle and gland cells, carrying information. As soon as their job is done, the body breaks them down and recycles them – live fast, die young. Once the neurotransmitter has reached its destination, it will attach itself to a receptor on its target cell, relay the message and get a response, including effects on mood and behaviour.

## gut feeling

The brain and the intestine might as well be married. This is a serious physical and biochemical relationship, where they communicate with each other, and is why the intestine is often referred to as the 'second brain'. The intestine is sensitive and highly influenced by what the brain is doing and this is entirely reciprocated. Anything from partying too hard or not eating well to taking antibiotics disrupts the intestinal microbiota, which can interfere with mood levels.

# we four, we happy four

Endorphins, dopamine, serotonin and oxytocin are all types of 'happy' chemicals that help reduce stress and pain in the body, increase pleasure and make us feel good.

### ▸ ENDORPHINS

Endorphins are masters at helping the body deal with pain and anxiety. Something as simple as laughter can actually trigger the brain to release them – even the anticipation of laughter prompts endorphin production, like meeting up with an incredibly funny friend or sending someone a hilarious meme. 'Runner's high', the feeling people get after vigorous exercise, is due to a surge in exhilarating endorphins.

### ▸ OXYTOCIN

Nicknamed the 'love hormone', oxytocin is a neurotransmitter that helps build intimacy, trust in relationships and bonding between mother and baby. It also gets released during social bonding – for example, when you hug someone or play with a friendly dog.

### ▸ SEROTONIN

Serotonin is made from the amino acid L-tryptophan, which the body turns into 5-HTP and then serotonin, meaning that a diet deficient in tryptophan will inhibit the production of serotonin. Approximately 95 per cent of serotonin is made by the small intestine's microbiota. It is involved in the regeneration of brain cells and also works as a brain neurotransmitter, balancing moods, feelings of satisfaction, happiness, optimism and the regulation of the circadian rhythm. This is why the digestive system can significantly affect moods and immunity.

### ▸ DOPAMINE

Dopamine will be released in response to an expected or experienced pleasure, telling the brain, 'We thoroughly enjoyed that – definitely do it again.'

# GABA – and relaaaaaaaax…

GABA is the brain's calming influence, facilitating communication between neurons and helping to suppress stress and anxiety. It serves a lot of different functions in the body, increasing feelings of relaxation, balancing moods, relieving pain and improving sleep. Interestingly, alcohol consumption can affect how GABA works in the body, as slurring and feeling socially disinhibited or sleepy are all partially the result of GABA's sedentary effects being increased. You can now add, 'It wasn't me, it was my amino acids,' to your list of excuses after a big night.

# noradrenaline – pay attention

The main neurotransmitter of the sympathetic nervous system, noradrenaline helps the brain's attention span, concentration and ability to remember. It plays an important role in the 'fight or flight' response by contracting muscles, increasing blood flow and heart rate, bringing the body into an acute state of awareness by sharpening the senses and increasing vigilance.

# disrupted neurotransmitters

Disrupted levels of neurotransmitters means signals don't get relayed, resulting in the actions or feelings they are responsible for being compromised, reduced or eliminated. Contributers include:

## ▸ DIET
The body needs the right materials, like amino acids, vitamins and minerals to make all of the brain's neurotransmitters. Impaired digestion and absorption and a diet that doesn't contain enough variety can reduce production.

## ▸ TOXINS
Neurotransmitter production and function are affected by alcohol, caffeine, prescription medication, recreational drugs and nicotine. These substances can boost neurotransmitter levels, tricking the body into feeling good, but this is only temporary, and a low mood may follow. Pesticides and heavy metals can also cause long-term damage to neurotransmitter behaviour.

## ▸ STRESS
It is natural for the body to experience periods of stress and its response is completely normal. Part of that process involves cortisol, which steals nutrients to support its increased production. What creates problems is when this response becomes chronic and fails to shut off and reset after a difficult situation has passed.

## ▸ GENETICS
Genetic predisposition can influence mental health. Some lucky people have a naturally cheery disposition because they happen to be able to generate higher levels of dopamine or serotonin, while the reverse is true for those who typically produce less.

## seasonal sadness

Seasonal affective disorder (SAD) is a type of depression brought on by a seasonally triggered chemical imbalance. Reduced daylight in winter can lead some people to experience a reduction in serotonin and an increase in the sleepy hormone melatonin, resulting in feelings of irritability, lethargy, lack of concentration, poor sleep and low mood.

# So what do we do?

It can be hard to find the motivation to improve a low mood when it has taken grip, but these are some gentle recommendations that can help the body begin to rebalance. It goes without saying that any clinical diagnosis needs professional assistance, whether that's medication or emotional support from a GP, trusted friends and family members.

## THREE IS THE MAGIC NUMBER

I have found that these nutrients are particularly good at addressing low moods and anxiety, supporting the body's natural ability to recover, rebalance and help the clouds to part.

### 1 TRYPTOPHAN + 5HTP = yay

Tryptophan is an amino acid precursor to 5-HTP, which the body then turns into serotonin and is found in certain foods. 5-HTP, on the other hand, has no dietary source, but can be taken in supplement form:

▸ *Tryptophan: poultry (chicken, turkey), eggs, cheese (parmesan, cheddar, mozzarella, gruyere), fish (halibut, salmon, trout, snapper, mackerel, haddock, cod), seeds (chia, sesame, pumpkin, sunflower, flax), peanuts, lentils, beans, tofu, oats, buckwheat.*

As tryptophan is found in high quantities in animal products, I suggest a 5-HTP supplement for vegans and vegetarians. However, this is not suitable for anyone being treated with prescribed medication for a mental health condition.

### 2 L-THEANINE – ommmmmm

L-theanine is a compound that increases levels of serotonin and GABA in the body, replacing feelings of stress and anxiety with a sense of calm. Its magic is in its ability to make us feel relaxed but not sleepy:

▸ *Tea leaves, particularly green tea. L-theanine is highly water-soluble, so when tea is prepared, nearly all of it dissolves from the leaves into the water (this does not include herbal teas because they're not made from tea leaves).*

*Start 5-HTP from a lower dose of 30–50mg, building up from there. Take for 2–3 months maximum, just to give the body a bit of a helping hand.*

*While I love green tea, you can avoid caffeine but get the benefits from L-theanine by taking it in supplement form.*

*Brain-boosting extra virgin olive oil and lemon juice is a far better option than sugary shop-bought dressings.*

*Tell life to calm down by taking GABA supplements if things are a bit stressy, starting with a smaller dose of 100mg (preferably in the evening) and increasing if necessary.*

## 3 GABA – DON'T WORRY, BE HAPPY

GABA relaxes the body and mind, reducing feelings of fear, stress and anxiety by attaching to proteins in the brain and producing a calming effect on the body. Some of these foods contain GABA, but they also help the body to synthesise it:

▸ *Fermented foods: kimchi, miso, tempeh, plain live yogurt, sauerkraut, kefir; cruciferous vegetables, soya beans, mushrooms, spinach, brown rice, peas, sweet potatoes.*

## ENDORPHINS – SWEAT IT OUT

As little as 30 minutes of physical activity or moderate exercise will release endorphins. This doesn't necessarily mean the gym, but a brisk walk, cycling instead of driving, using the stairs instead of the lift, or getting off the bus or tube early and walking the rest of the way all count.

*Group exercise may be better for those experiencing a low mood. Not only is it easier to stick to (joint commitments are harder to get out of), it can take the pressure off self-motivation if there is someone else joining in. Aim to do some form of exercise 3–4 times a week for at least 30 minutes.*

## CHEERFUL FATS FOR THE BRAIN

As the brain itself is nearly 60 per cent fat, fatty acids are crucial to how it functions, protecting against inflammation, supporting cell membrane integrity and neurotransmitter communication. Low-fat diets can cause all kinds of problems – for example, cholesterol levels that drop too low may result in serotonin activity being reduced – and no one wants that.

It's important to have a balance of fats in the diet and when it comes to cognitive function and mental health, there are two clear favourites – monounsaturated and polyunsaturated fatty acids.

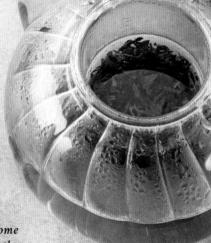

*Fish oil is incredibly important for a healthy brain, but some supplements can leave a fishy aftertaste. Keeping them in the freezer is a cunning way to reduce this effect.*

*I often recommend olives as a snack. Tapenade is great as a dip, and don't forget to add them to martinis. (And you wondered why 007 is the world's greatest spy. COINCIDENCE? I think not.)*

*Calling all those who don't like fish: in addition to including omega-3 through sources like nuts and seeds, take supplements extracted from algae, which is what the fish will have eaten to get their omega-3 in the first place.*

## MY MONO-HEROES
### Avocados

Apart from being a great source of monounsaturated fat, avocados contain choline, which increases levels of serotonin and dopamine. They're also packed with cysteine and vitamin B5, both of which assist with concentration and energy levels.

### Extra virgin olive oil

Rich in antioxidants, this oil keeps the brain powered up, while helping to improve its memory and the capacity to learn. It provides amazing support through the ageing process, helping to keep the brain sprightly:

▶ *Other mono-fats: peanut and sesame oils, olives, nuts (almonds, peanuts, hazelnuts, pecans, macadamia, cashews), seeds (pumpkin, sesame, hemp, sunflower).*

## MY POLY-HEROES
### Oily fish

Oily fish and shellfish are packed to the gills (literally) with omega-3, an essential fatty acid which increases blood flow to the brain, improves cognition and helps balance moods:

▶ *Salmon, mackerel, sardines, herring, anchovies, trout, tuna, halibut, mussels, oysters, prawns, clams, crayfish.*

### Nuts and seeds

Nuts and seeds are great brain food, as they are good sources of omega-3 and vitamin E (which helps reduce oxidative stress linked to ageing):

▶ *Nuts – walnuts, almonds, cashews, Brazil nuts, hazelnuts, peanuts.*
▶ *Seeds – sunflower, pumpkin, flax, hemp, sesame, chia.*

## PROTEINS

When digested, proteins become amino acids, which are needed to synthesise neurotransmitters, including endorphins, noradrenaline, dopamine and serotonin. Protein is the building contractor for all these mood-regulating chemicals. Unlike builders, protein makes you happy. Include a protein source at every meal:

▶ *Animal sources – lean meat (chicken, turkey, red meat), fish (salmon, mackerel, cod, sea bass, haddock, tuna), shellfish (prawns, clams, crab, crayfish), dairy products (milk, yogurt, kefir), egg.*
▶ *Plant sources – nuts (almonds, cashews, hazelnuts, walnuts, peanuts), seeds (pumpkin, sunflower, hemp, flax, chia), lentils, chickpeas, beans.*

*Nuts and seeds bring a delicious crunch to pretty much everything. Blitzed up, they can be used instead of breadcrumbs on chicken or fish, as well as added to soups, salads, porridge, pudding… I could go on.*

## CAFFEINE AND BRAIN FOCUS

Like many things in life, caffeine is not straightforward. But in the context of brain function, it can actually be beneficial. Caffeine blocks the function of adenosine, a compound in the brain associated with sleepiness. Caffeinated drinks like coffee and green tea are also both potent sources of antioxidants. However, it doesn't agree with everyone and is best avoided by those experiencing problems with sleeping, stress or anxiety.

## DARK CHOCOLATE

Apart from benefiting the liver and supporting sleep, dark chocolate can also contribute to cognitive function. The brain becomes increasingly vulnerable to oxidative stress through ageing and the cacao in dark chocolate contains flavonoids – antioxidants that can help tackle it.

Flavonoids are also believed to assist in the growth of neurons and blood vessels in the parts of the brain associated with memory and learning, as well as stimulating the brain's blood flow and improving its plasticity. No wonder we love to curl up with a big bar of chocolate. It's literally making us cleverer.

## A LITTLE NOTE ON ALCOHOL

When life gets stressful, it's not uncommon to think, 'I could do with a drink.' One goes down quickly, two starts to feel relaxing, three is now really oiling the wheels – and so on. However, alcohol suppresses the central nervous system and this results in fluctuating moods. The bit that feels good not only doesn't last, but also comes at a price. Many of us understand the need to drink in moderation, but I also know that it's an individual decision and that boozy nights are a part of life for some people.

*My own personal approach is to drink lots of water between glasses of wine. It's surprisingly filling – a cheap trick that means you end up drinking less booze. Not always, but sometimes. Worth a try.*

## LIGHT THERAPY

Those experiencing the effects of SAD are usually advised to take up exercise, especially something that can be done outdoors during daylight hours. Another option is light therapy or phototherapy, which involves 30 minutes of daily exposure to an artificial light source that is stronger than daylight. It works through the eyes, not the skin, and the effects can be pretty instant. However, it's normal to need a few days or weeks to see an improvement.

*Switch a SAD light on intermittently during the winter months to boost light exposure. It also works as a lamp. Useful.*

### Superhero supplements

- 5-HTP
- L-theanine
- GABA
- Probiotics
- Adaptogens (individually or combined) – ginkgo biloba, ashwagandha, maca, rhodiola
- Omega-3
- Vitamin B complex

# 9/

## the heart
*and* lungs

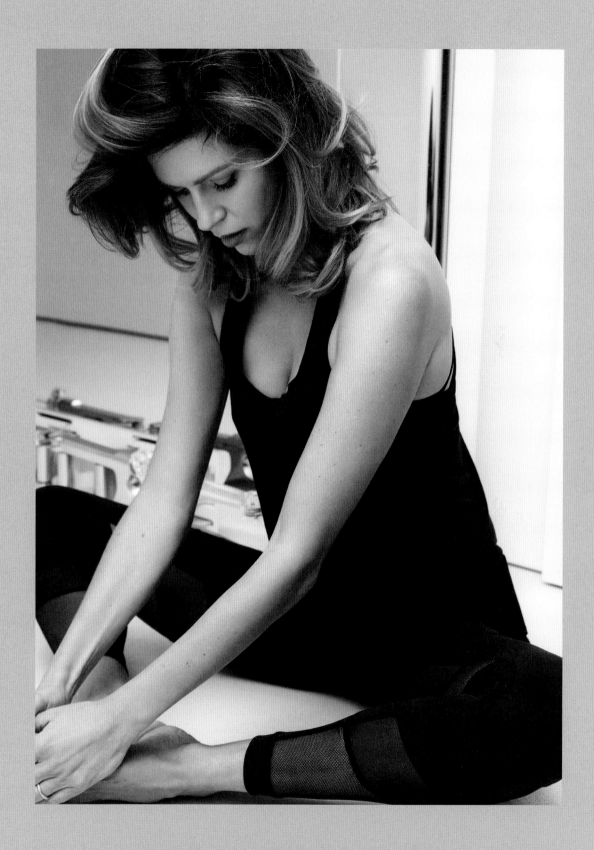

*do you* ...

☐ often get stressed?

☐ feel you are overweight?

☐ have a history of high blood pressure or cholesterol in the family?

☐ find you're easily susceptible to respiratory infections?

☐ smoke?

The heart and lungs operate as two systems in the body, but they are intricately linked. Their specialist subjects are supplying oxygen to and removing carbon dioxide from the body in a constantly running cycle.

# breathing and oxygen exchange

Oxygen is critical for cell function. They cannot survive without it, so in order for the body to acquire and process it properly, it needs to go through three stages. Ventilation is the act of inhaling and allowing oxygen to travel through the lungs. Diffusion is when oxygen passes into the blood. Finally, perfusion is where oxygen travels into the tissues and cells.

The respiratory system balances oxygen and carbon dioxide levels within the body's organs, tissues and blood and will respond to any changes as they occur in order to maintain homeostasis. During exercise, our breathing rate will increase in order to raise oxygen intake, while the heart pumps faster to deliver the oxygen to the muscles. About a fifth of the air we breathe is made up of oxygen, of which the body uses only a tiny amount. The rest is exhaled as waste via the lungs through the simple act of breathing.

*To give your body a quick, hearty oxygen boost, drink a glass of water, as lungs need hydration to work effectively. Take a brisk walk and have an iron-rich snack, like a slice of turkey or some dried apricots and figs.*

# the beat of the heart

The heart pumps oxygenated blood all over the body, which facilitates the distribution of nutrients, immune cells and hormones. It also transports carbon dioxide and other metabolic waste from the kidneys, lungs and liver, working to regulate body temperature in conjunction with the hypothalamus.

The number of times the heart contracts is how the heart rate is measured. The average adult in a resting state will have 60–100 beats per minute – that's roughly 100,000 times a day. The more fit someone is, the lower their heart rate.

The volume of blood pumped around the body in 1 minute is known as cardiac output and the speed at which it travels is controlled by the rate at which the heart contracts. This output will directly affect how efficiently nutrients and oxygen are delivered and waste is removed. Many different factors can affect the heart rate, including exercise, excitement, fear, illness, sleep and rest.

The autonomic nervous system is what unconsciously regulates the heart rate and contractility. When the parasympathetic nervous system (the body's 'rest or digest' state) is active, the heart rate is steady and methodical. When the sympathetic nervous system has been activated ('fight or flight'), it sends adrenaline and noradrenaline to the heart to speed it up, so that blood will pump faster and the body will become more alert. The body is brilliantly able to respond to these changes, allowing for minimal disruption.

# the transportation system

Like a private tube network, the cardiovascular system contains vessels of varying sizes and functions that carry blood all over the body in a constantly moving cycle.

**ARTERIES** (excluding the pulmonary and umbilical arteries) – these vessels carry oxygenated blood away from the heart to all parts of the body. Their walls are made of three sturdy layers in order to cope with the pressure of the blood flow from the heart.

**VEINS** – these vessels transport deoxygenated blood from the body's peripheries to the heart and on to the lungs. Their blood pressure is lower, which means their walls don't need to be as thick.

**CAPILLARIES** – the smallest of the vessels. Capillaries are incredibly thin and permeable, which allows for the quick and easy diffusion of substances like oxygen and nutrients into tissues and organs.

**GP** *tip*

*Crush or soak plant sterols like flax seeds before adding them to cereal, porridge or yogurt, as this increases the body's ability to absorb them. Their omega-3 content and cholesterol-balancing properties are fantastic for cardiovascular health.*

# Blood

Blood is the body's river transportation. This highly specialised fluid, which is around 80 per cent water, is comprised of the below. Blood has numerous jobs, which include transporting oxygen, carbon dioxide, immune cells, nutrients and hormones, clotting wounds to prevent infection, distributing heat and carrying waste to the liver and kidneys to be processed out of the body.

## ▶ Red blood cells (RBC)
RBCs are the most common type of blood cell and around 2 million are produced every second. They're shaped a bit like an indented doughnut with no hole, which cleverly increases the surface area of the cell, facilitating the speedy absorption and release of substances like oxygen and carbon dioxide, as well as enabling them to move easily through blood vessels.

### Haemoglobin
*This iron-containing protein accounts for 95 per cent of a red blood cell's structure and is the gentle hand-holding agent that enables gases to be transported throughout the body. Each RBC contains around 270 million haemoglobin molecules capable of carrying four oxygen molecules each.*

## ▶ Platelets
These tiny cells are called to action when a blood vessel is damaged. Platelets respond to the alert signal sent out when an injury occurs and rush to the scene to stop any bleeding by forming clots. This is called adhesion.

## ▶ White blood cells (WBC)
WBCs form the body's immune system. Their job is to patrol via the bloodstream looking for pathogens, engulfing low-level threats and triggering specialised responses to viruses and harmful bacteria. They account for about 1 per cent of blood, but what they lack in numbers, they make up for in impact. More mind-blowing facts on page 34.

## ▶ Plasma
Plasma is the fluid element of the blood and its largest component, coming in at around 55 per cent. In isolation, plasma is a pale-yellow colour that is around 90 per cent water. Its job is to carry all the elements within blood around the body and to assist in removing waste.

## ▶ Blood pressure
In order for blood to be pumped from the heart to the peripheries, its pressure must be high enough to overcome any kind of resistance, like blockages or narrowed arteries.

## THE BLOOD-BRAIN BARRIER
The body is so protective of the central nervous system that it surrounds it with a semi-permeable border of cells called the blood-brain barrier. This system means that glucose, oxygen and nutrients can pass through, but not pathogens and toxins. That's why commonplace infections don't make the brain ill. Getting in to see *Hamilton* is easier.

# know your lipids

Triglycerides and cholesterol are fatty substances known as lipids. Triglycerides act as the main source of long-term stored energy, while cholesterol is a waxy substance that is used to build healthy cell walls. Neither can travel in water on their own, so the body attaches them to lipoproteins, their own speed boats, in order to distribute them via the bloodstream.

## triglycerides

Triglycerides are made from three fatty acids and glycerol (a form of glucose) and are used by the body to generate energy when the short-term storage in the liver and muscles is running low. They can also be obtained through diet and are mostly found in meat, dairy products and oils.

## cholesterol

Cholesterol is not actually a fat, but a wax-like substance. Like triglycerides, it is both synthesised in the liver and also found in animal fats. Cholesterol may have had bad press over the years, but it plays important structural and functional roles in the body. Around only 20 per cent of the body's cholesterol levels come from the diet and the rest is made by the liver. This means reducing amounts of dietary cholesterol alone tends to make little difference, because it may only result in the liver generating more to maintain homeostasis. Genetics are more likely to influence cholesterol levels by potentially preventing the removal of excess amounts from the blood or allowing the liver to produce too much. That doesn't mean it can't be managed in other ways; obesity, smoking and alcohol can also raise cholesterol levels and all of those can be changed.

---

### WHY WE NEED CHOLESTEROL

▶ **Cell membranes** – every cell in the body needs cholesterol. Not only is it used to shape and build cell walls, it influences their capability, from interpreting hormone signals to the absorption of molecules like nutrients.

▶ **Steroid hormones** – cholesterol is a precursor for androgens, oestrogens and progestogens. These are key messengers which follow signals from the brain and deliver information to organs and tissues.

▶ **Bile salts** – one of the components of bile salts, cholesterol is produced in the liver and stored in the gallbladder. Bile is secreted during digestion to assist the breakdown of fats.

▶ **Vitamin D** – cholesterol in skin cells is a precursor to vitamin D3, which gets synthesised when cells come into contact with sunlight. Vitamin D plays several important roles, like keeping bones, teeth and muscles strong and the immune system healthy.

# lipoproteins

Most of us are familiar with the terms 'good' and 'bad' cholesterol, but it is actually its lipoprotein carrier that will determine its status. This is decided by the amount of cholesterol that the lipoprotein is transporting. The lower its saturation, the more it is considered to be bad or unhealthy because its lighter load means there is more cholesterol circulating in the blood. A cholesterol test is actually measuring the lipoprotein's cholesterol uptake, not the cholesterol itself.

### LOW-DENSITY LIPOPROTEIN (LDL)

No thank you. LDL ('bad' cholesterol) transports cholesterol around the body from the liver to peripheral tissues. Too much of it can lead to a build-up of 'plaque', which can narrow and harden artery walls, making it more difficult for blood to flow.

### HIGH-DENSITY LIPOPROTEIN (HDL)

Yes please. HDL ('good' cholesterol) absorbs excess cholesterol and carries it back to the liver to be used in the production of the gall bladder's bile or packaged up for excretion. This process can help lower the risk of blocked arteries and heart disease.

*Another reason to pay your respects to soluble fibre: it attaches itself to cholesterol in order to regulate how much the body absorbs. Clever. Add psyllium husk to a green juice or smoothie to ensure a healthy intake.*

# what can go wrong?

While we might all consider ourselves to be young, dynamic and vital with health(!), cardio-respiratory conditions are not just for the old and overweight. It's never too early to start being conscious (in a non-hysterical way) about looking after these amazing mechanisms in the body.

## a hassled heart

Conditions that impact the cardiovascular system are unlikely to appear as one single problem. Usually there are several components that arrive, arms linked, and may lead to health issues. Even though genetic predisposition almost always plays a role, we know that when it comes to problems with the heart, diet and lifestyle are also significant culprits.

*Losing excess weight is a powerful way to protect the heart. It's been shown to reduce elevated blood pressure and high glucose levels, lower cholesterol and improve insulin resistance – and the good news is, it's possible for everyone to achieve.*

## HIGH BLOOD PRESSURE

Also known as hypertension, an increase in blood pressure can be due to the narrowing or hardening of the artery walls, which will trigger the heart to increase blood pressure in order to get through these restrictions.

## HIGH CHOLESTEROL AND EXCESSIVE TRIGLYCERIDES

Cholesterol is incredibly important for the body but it walks a tightrope, with high levels of LDL cholesterol capable of causing significant damage. Diet, lifestyle and genetics can all influence how cholesterol behaves in the body and while it's not easy to change hereditary impact, it is possible to assist in eliminating surplus cholesterol in other ways. Excess calories, alcohol or sugar are also turned into triglycerides and because this then creates an overflow, the body stores them in fat cells for later use. They are then released by hormones for energy between meals. If more calories are eaten than are burned, this can lead to weight gain. High levels of triglycerides from a sugary diet can also contribute to the narrowing of artery walls, which can result in high blood pressure and inflammation.

## ATHEROSCLEROSIS

Hardened, narrowed or blocked arteries can make it difficult for blood to flow easily, which increases pressure, overworking the heart and putting blood vessels under strain. This can lead to bits of plaque or clots breaking away into the bloodstream, potentially causing damage like heart attacks, strokes or aneurysms.

# metabolic syndrome

Metabolic syndrome is a combination of conditions – high blood sugar levels, increased blood pressure, excess abdominal fat, high amounts of triglycerides and abnormal cholesterol levels – where at least three out of five are experienced at the same time. Ageing, ethnicity, excessive weight and diabetes can all contribute. Experiencing one of these conditions on its own is not an indicator of metabolic syndrome, but it might suggest an increased risk of illness. Metabolic syndrome also has close links to insulin resistance, which can turn into type 2 diabetes.

# excess bodyweight

Being overweight can put a serious strain on many systems within the body. Too much fat around the abdomen is a strong indicator of cardiovascular risk. The most effective way to find out if it's time to lose weight is by doing the waist–hip ratio test. A healthy result for men is 0.9 or less and for women, it's 0.85 or less.

### THE WHR TEST (USE A TAPE MEASURE)
- Stand up straight, relax and exhale.
- Measure above the belly button around the smallest part of the waist.
- Measure around the widest part of the hips.
- Divide the waist measurement by the hip measurement. The result is your WHR.

# upsetting the lungs

The lungs are constantly filtering everything the body inhales. In addition to chronic conditions, bacteria and viruses like colds and flu are always loitering with intent but get worse in winter as people congregate indoors in closer proximity. These infections can spread very easily, travelling through coughs and sneezes as droplets are sprayed through the air and they can survive on surfaces for hours.

## ▸ ASTHMA

Asthma is a chronic lung condition that affects hundreds of millions of people all over the world. Asthma attacks cause the lining of the bronchial tubes to become swollen and narrowed, producing too much mucus. This leads to breathlessness, wheezing, coughing and a tight chest, as air flow to the lungs is inhibited. Asthma is normally the result of a genetic condition and/or exposure to inhaled environmental irritants, like dust mites, pollution, animal fur, pollen, moulds, tobacco smoke or chemicals.

## ▸ FLU

A lot of people refer to a bad cold as flu and while the symptoms are similar, this condition is caused by the influenza virus and can develop into a serious illness. Flu is usually experienced as a fever, chills, muscle aches, headaches and tiredness, as well as a sore throat, cough and runny nose. For most people, flu usually means feeling pretty unwell in bed for anything from a few days to a couple of weeks; for others, it has the potential to turn into bacterial pneumonia and other infections, which may require hospitalisation.

## ▸ BRONCHITIS

Bronchitis is the swelling of the bronchi, the air passages in the lungs. The pathogen will inflame these tubes, fill them with sticky mucus and compromise air flow, which the lungs will try to dislodge through coughing. There are two types: acute starts to improve in 2–3 weeks, whilst chronic bronchitis means symptoms of a cough and mucus are ongoing, persisting for at least 3 consecutive months.

## ▸ PNEUMONIA

Viruses, bacteria and fungi can all cause pneumonia, which is where one or both of the lungs becomes inflamed. Germs infect the lungs' tiny but critical air sacs, which interferes with oxygen getting into the bloodstream and creates breathing difficulties. As well as shortness of breath, the swelling may trigger a fever, cough and chest pain. Pneumonia has the potential to become dangerous and can require medical attention.

## ▸ THE COMMON COLD

There are more than 200 types of virus or bacteria that can lead to the misery of a streaming nose and watery eyes, but it's the rhinovirus that is responsible for over 50 per cent of colds. They are the most common viral infection humans can pick up.

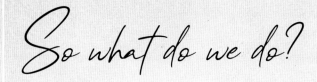

# So what do we do?

## THE MEDITERRANEAN DIET

There is not much that isn't fantastic about the Mediterranean way of life, especially when it comes to diet. It takes inspiration from the foods that are traditionally eaten in Italy, Spain and Greece where the focus is on simple ingredients, simply prepared – fresh, locally sourced vegetables, fish, wholegrains, healthy fats like olive oil, nuts and seeds, all washed down with a glass of good red wine. This is a diet comprised of elements that are particularly good for healthy, happy hearts.

### Fibre

Fibre is a carbohydrate the body cannot absorb and a multi-faceted champion fighter when it comes to protecting the heart. As little as 5–10g (1–2 teaspoons) of soluble fibre a day can reduce LDL levels, as fibre attaches itself to cholesterol in the intestinal tract, preventing it from getting absorbed into the bloodstream. Fibre also lowers blood pressure and makes the body feel fuller after eating, helping to balance blood sugar levels and reduce weight gain and its associated health risks to the heart:

▸ *Cereals (bran, porridge oats), grains (barley, brown rice, quinoa, buckwheat), vegetables (spinach, broccoli, Brussels sprouts, carrots, green beans), beans, pulses, fruit (pears, apples, prunes).*
▸ *Flax seeds, psyllium and glucomannan are fantastic sources of fibre.*

### Plant sterols/phytosterols

As we all know, HDL cholesterol is the goodie because it helps the body get rid of LDL, which is the baddie. Plant sterols (or phytosterols) are phytochemicals that are similar in structure to cholesterol. Along with HDL, they help manage LDL levels and reduce the risk of heart disease by competing with cholesterol for absorption in the digestive tract:

▸ *Nuts (almonds, walnuts, pistachios, cashews, pecans), flax seeds, wholegrains (rye, wheat), vegetables (broccoli, corn, sprouts, carrots, red onions), fruit (blueberries, avocado, strawberries), olive oil, beans, pulses.*

*Instead of ordering white rice with a takeaway, I always make my own quinoa or brown rice. Okay, full disclosure, I don't even do that. I heat it up from a pre-cooked pouch. Done in 2 minutes. The whole point of takeaways is to do zero work.*

*While dietary sources are usually preferable, plant sterols also come in supplement form, making it very easy to top up levels of this clever cholesterol impersonator.*

**GP** *tip* → This is a short story entitled 'Eat More Fish'. The end.

## Fats

Fat is an essential part of a healthy diet. Without it, the body cannot absorb fat-soluble vitamins, such as A, D and E. While some fats are critical for the body to function properly, others are less so (see page 18). This is how they link specifically to cardiovascular health.

Trans fatty acids are the least good. Found in many manufactured and fried foods, like cakes, biscuits, doughnuts and margarine, they can increase levels of LDL cholesterol, without doing the same for HDL. Saturated fats fall more into the middle of the Venn diagram, as they're neither particularly good nor particularly bad. Found in fatty cuts of meat, like lamb and beef, dairy, lard and tropical oils, they are best managed by making sure they are well balanced with better fats, which leads us to monounsaturated and polyunsaturated, both of which are at the top of the tree. Monounsaturated fats can decrease levels of LDL cholesterol and lower the risk of cardiovascular disease:

▸ *Olive oil, avocados, nuts (almonds, cashews, peanuts, pistachios), seeds (pumpkin, sunflower), eggs.*

The real stars are the polyunsaturated fats, which contain powerful anti-inflammatory properties (very relevant for heart health) and which lower triglycerides levels, blood pressure and the risk of forming blood clots:

▸ *Oily fish (mackerel, herring, salmon, trout, sardines, tuna), shellfish (mussels, oysters, crab), nuts (walnuts, almonds, macadamia, hazelnuts, pecans), seeds (pumpkin, sunflower, hemp, chia, flax).*

## Red wine and resveratrol

Red wine contains a plant compound called resveratrol, which has antioxidant capabilities and is believed to help protect the lining of the heart's blood vessels and lower blood pressure. Resveratrol comes from the skin and seeds of red grapes, which is why it's found in red wine. The plot thickens, though. Along with resveratrol, it has been suggested that low levels of alcohol increase HDL, reduce LDL and prevent a build-up of cholesterol, as well as protect against blood clots. Before you open the windows and start shouting, 'WINE IS MEDICINE, EVERYONE!' this is beneficial only when alcohol is drunk in moderation – for reasons we are all aware of. It's really about finding a balance, where the good elements are not completely overwhelmed by the bad and that is a fine line to walk:

▸ *Nuts (pistachios, peanuts), red wine (Pinot noir, Merlot), red grapes, cocoa, berries (blueberries, cranberries).*

**GP** *tip* → Taking a resveratrol supplement delivers high quantities of this amazing antioxidant into the body without the risk of a hangover.

## GET A MOVE ON

There's nothing that makes the heart happier than a healthy dose of regular physical activity. It strengthens the heart muscle, keeps weight down and helps protect against high cholesterol, blood sugar and blood pressure. Aerobic exercise helps to boost circulation and maintain a healthy blood pressure and heart rate, as well as balanced blood sugar levels. Resistance training helps to reduce excess body fat, build muscle and improve the overall composition of the body. Regularly practising both these forms of exercise can also help increase HDL and lower LDL cholesterol levels.

- ▸ *Aerobic exercise means increasing the heart and breathing rate, getting the blood pumping and making the body break a sweat. This could be anything from brisk walking, cycling, swimming, running or playing a sport like tennis – aim for 30 minutes, 3–5 days a week.*
- ▸ *Resistance training means working out with dumbbells, hand weights, barbells, resistance bands or gym weight machines, as well as exercises that include push-ups, squats and chin-ups – ideally twice a week.*

 *Take the stairs instead of the escalator and walk or cycle instead of driving. You know you want to.*

 *Chia seeds are rich in omega-3 and magnesium. Soak them in yogurt overnight and eat with berries. A hearty (sorry) breakfast.*

## STRESS LESS

The body responds to stress with well over 1,000 biochemical reactions. While stress is a normal part of life, an elevated blood pressure and speeding heart rate are not meant to be experienced on a regular basis or over extended periods of time. Chronic stress-related inflammation has been linked to plaque formation in the arteries, which can lead to blood clots. It can also affect the consistency of the blood, making it stickier and increasing the risk of heart-related complications. Chronic stress is incredibly draining and can lead to increased blood sugar, cholesterol and triglyceride levels, all of which can cause problems for the heart. There are many different ways to address stress (see page 91), but they generally include:

- ▸ *Improving bedtime habits to get a better night's sleep.*
- ▸ *Eating more essential fatty acids, which helps to balance hormone levels.*
- ▸ *Including more magnesium, the body's natural relaxant, in the diet.*
- ▸ *Supplementing adaptogen herbs to support adrenal function.*
- ▸ *Exercising regularly to generate endorphins, the body's happy chemicals.*
- ▸ *Consuming more fibre to ensure used hormones are efficiently eliminated.*

 *Mash together some avocado, chilli, lime juice and a dash of olive oil with pumpkin seeds and have on toasted rye bread. Fibre, magnesium and vitamin E – your heart's dream breakfast.*

## CHALLENGE THE LUNGS

We don't ever really think about exercising the lungs, but like all parts of the body, they need it. Breathing in and out as normal isn't enough of a workout for the lungs on its own. They need help to flush out toxins from pollutants found in the environment, dust, allergens and smoke. Most unconscious breathing is shallow and from the chest, so breathing deeply from the diaphragm helps blow away the cobwebs (the lower abdomen should rise and fall).

▸ *Inhale slowly for a count of four. Exhale slowly for a count of eight. Whatever the length, the exhalation needs to be twice as long as the inhalation.*

 *This breathing technique can be done on the move/while your pets are fighting/when the dishwasher breaks – anywhere, any time.*

 *Who knew baths could increase oxygen levels? The pressure and warmth of the water can expand breathing and lung capacity.*

## NATURE'S MEDICINE CABINET
### Vitamins D and E

Not only can vitamin D help support the immune system, it can also contribute to reducing inflammation in the airways. In fact, low levels of vitamin D can increase the risk of having an asthma attack:

▸ *Oily fish (salmon, trout, mackerel, sardines, tuna), egg yolks, red meat, liver, mushrooms and obviously sunshine.*

Vitamin E may help relieve asthmatic symptoms, like coughing and wheezing, by reducing inflammation:

▸ *Nuts (Brazil nuts, almonds, hazelnuts), seeds (sunflower, pine nuts), vegetables (Swiss chard, kale, broccoli, spinach, avocado, butternut squash), kiwi fruit, olive oil.*

 *Vitamin D is essential for heart and lung health and while the sun is its most powerful source, supplements are a really easy way to keep levels topped up during winter, particularly between October and March.*

### Magnesium

The great natural relaxer, magnesium can help reduce air restriction in the bronchioles of the lungs, as well as decrease inflammation. Improved lung function has been linked to higher magnesium levels, while for those who suffer with lung problems, symptoms can become worse when their magnesium levels are low. It's also one of the most important minerals for heart health, reducing spasms and blood pressure.

It helps the heart to relax by countering the effects of calcium – which makes the heart contract – thereby helping to maintain a healthy heart beat:

▸ *Leafy greens (Swiss chard, spinach, kale, collard greens), seeds (chia, pumpkin, flax, sesame), nuts (almonds, Brazil nuts, cashews), beans, lentils, chickpeas, fish (tuna, mackerel), grains (brown rice, quinoa, buckwheat), dark chocolate.*

*The heart, the lungs, the whole body – loves magnesium in large amounts. This doesn't mean having to swallow down a lot of pills, as it also comes in powder form, oil spray and bath flakes, so take your pick.*

## Carotenoids

These plant pigments are found in brightly coloured vegetables and fruit and are very beneficial for the lungs. For example, tomatoes contain high levels of lycopene, a carotenoid antioxidant that is linked to the reduction of inflammation in the lungs:

▶ *Vegetables (pumpkins, butternut squash, romaine lettuce, red peppers, carrots, sweet potatoes, kale, collard greens, Swiss chard), fruit (mangoes, cantaloupe melon, apricots).*

*Ketchup – but not as you know it. Swap it for lycopene-rich tomato purée, which is naturally sweet and not rammed with artificial sugars – unlike its shop-bought nemesis, which has zero nutritional value.*

## Superhero supplements

### Heart
- Plant sterols
- Magnesium
- Glucomannan/Psyllium
- CoQ10
- Omega-3
- Curcumin

### Lungs
- Quercetin
- N-acetyl cysteine
- Vitamin D
- Omega-3
- Curcumin
- Magnesium

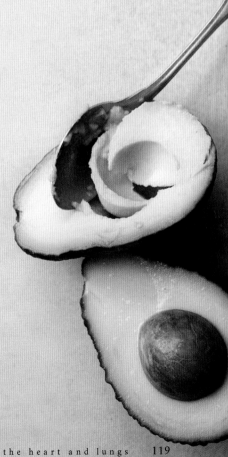

# 10/

## vital energy

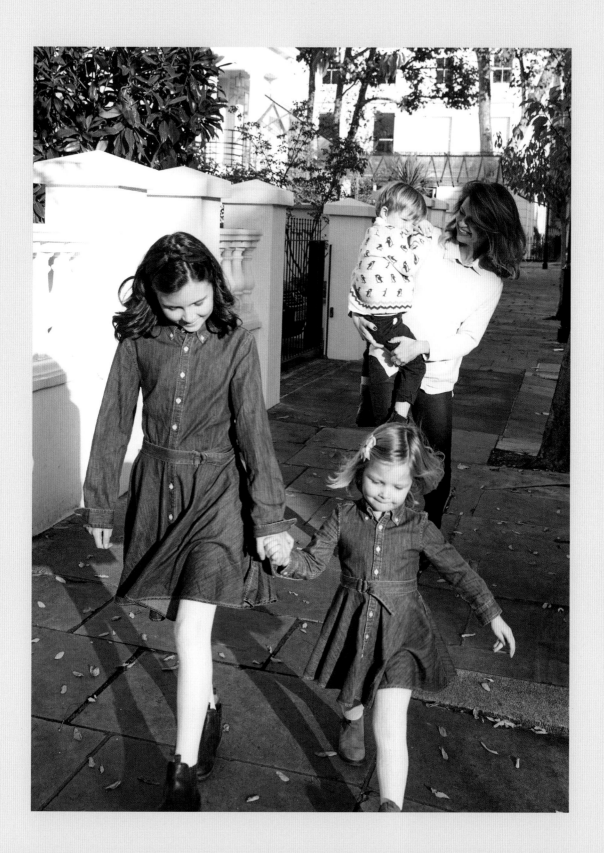

☐ regularly experience energy dips throughout the day?

☐ normally crave carbohydrates, sugary foods and caffeinated drinks?

☐ feel excessively hungry mid-morning and mid-afternoon?

☐ often feel tired?

☐ regularly have mood swings?

# why do we need energy?

There is nothing the body can do without energy. It fuels each and every function, from moving and growing to generating heat, keeping the heart beating, regulating the body's metabolism and enabling the lungs to breathe. The body even needs energy to do nothing. In a resting state, the brain consumes, on average, 20 per cent of the body's energy and even uses it to sleep.

## how does the body produce energy?

Every cell in the body requires energy in order to do its job effectively. The body begins the process of producing energy from the macronutrients (carbohydrates, fats and proteins) it consumes. While these all provide some degree of fuel, carbohydrates are the primary source and are found in vegetables, fruit, grains, legumes and dairy.

Carbohydrates are broken down into simple sugars like glucose, absorbed into the bloodstream and carried to the body's cells. Glucose begins its conversion through a process called glycolysis and is transported to the cell's mitochondria (its battery). This triggers another series of chemical reactions called the Krebs cycle, where the glucose converts into ATP (adenosine triphosphate), which is the unit of energy the body can now use. All this, just from eating a sandwich. Who knew?

Any leftover glucose that has been absorbed but not used goes through a process called glycogenesis, where the glucose is turned into glycogen and stored in liver and muscle cells. Should its cupboards become full, the liver cunningly converts glucose into triglycerides and sends it to adipose tissue for long-term storage.

Now would be a good moment to point out that there's nothing wrong with a bit of fat – in fact, we need it, particularly women – but when more is accumulated than used, it can lead to weight gain. In an ideal world, there would be a perfect equilibrium between the amount of energy the body generates and the amount it uses, with a little bit put away for emergencies (like running away from lions/screaming children, etc).

If the body hasn't been fed for a few hours, the muscles will turn to their own banked glycogen. The liver also begins to break down its glycogen stores, releasing it as glucose into the bloodstream to maintain a stable flow of energy. However, it can only manage this for approximately 10 hours before its personal reserves run low, when the body will then start to break down the triglycerides it put away in fat cells. The more active the body is, the quicker it will get through the glycogen reserves in the muscles and liver before moving on to fat.

# energy and blood sugar balance

Different foods contain different levels of sugars, which are absorbed into the bloodstream at different rates. The trick is to make sure a variety of macronutrients get represented on the plate. Carbohydrate-heavy food can cause a surge of sugars to rush into the bloodstream, while protein and fats, along with fibre, make their entrance at a more leisurely pace. If carbohydrates are eaten along with protein and fat, their sugars are absorbed more slowly in a calm, dignified manner. This is why eating carbohydrates on their own is not a good idea as the body will have got on the wild ride that is a sugar spike. 'YESSSSS,' it might find itself thinking after a doughnut, 'I feel GREAT.' That won't last – because what goes up, must come down. 'OH,' it'll think soon afterwards, 'I suddenly feel QUITE TIRED, GRUMPY, ANXIOUS and I am CRAVING MORE SUGAR.' Being deranged on sugar has its moments, but it is far better to aim for a slow, steady supply of energy through balanced meal composition and eating regularly, in order to avoid the rush and subsequent crash.

## the role of insulin

How does glucose actually get into the cells? It needs the help of insulin, a hormone produced by the pancreas. Insulin acts like a key, opening the cell's door, allowing the glucose to enter and be converted into energy. This happens a few times a day, depending on when, what and how much we eat and if it is balanced. Problems arise when the bloodstream is regularly flooded with lots of sugar. The liver, muscles and fat tissue start to ignore the signal from insulin to take glucose out of the blood and absorb it into the cells. As a result, the body is pushed to produce more insulin, exhausting the beta cells in the pancreas that secrete it. This is known as insulin resistance and, untreated, may lead to type 2 diabetes.

*Hands up if you drink coffee or tea on an empty stomach. Is that you? (It's so you, isn't it?). Caffeine stimulates the release of glucose into the bloodstream, causing sugar spikes, so try to have it with a balanced snack.*

# the rollercoaster of energy highs and lows

Energy dips happen for two reasons. It may be that the last meal eaten was not balanced or the gap between meals has been too long, causing blood sugar levels to drop and cravings to surge. This is how blood sugar imbalance leads to unhealthy choices. A similar thing is happening if hunger pangs start to rumble two hours after a meal. This is usually a sign that not enough protein, fat or fibre was included, as without them, the energy produced by any carbohydrates eaten wears off too quickly.

*The best way to eat fruit, especially the super-sweet tropical kind, is with a portion of protein, like nuts, seeds or live yogurt, as it slows down the sugar release, preventing spikes and dips.*

# energy and stress

The acute stress response is the body's way of keeping itself safe by preparing it to run from the perceived threat. It does this through an endocrine response that heightens alertness, suppresses the appetite and releases glucose from glycogen stores as an energy boost. Now a quick getaway can be made. If this stress response continues, though, it will lead to chronic stress. Unfortunately, the modern world and all its stressors has meant that a response designed for emergencies is stimulated on a regular basis.

Chronic stress behaves slightly differently to acute stress. The body releases the hormone cortisol, which actually increases appetite. When stress persists, the body is under constant demand to secrete cortisol, which can lead to all kinds of imbalances and also weight gain as it builds up reserves of adipose tissue. A constant stream of cortisol will also negatively impact energy levels. Nutrients are redirected from their normal day jobs to support the excess amount of cortisol being produced. Magnesium and B vitamins, which are among the nutrients specifically needed to create energy, are depleted, leaving the body feeling exhausted.

# energy and sleep

Decreased levels of glucose are another reason the body may feel low in energy. At the risk of sounding like Captain Obvious, sleeping badly will also have an impact. While the body is asleep, the brain performs some important overnight housekeeping. A large supply of ATP is delivered to the areas of the brain that are the most active during waking hours. This surge of cellular energy helps replenish those depleted regions, so that they are restored and ready to go again when the body wakes up. Disrupted sleep interferes with this process, meaning the brain is working at a reduced capacity before the day has even started.

*Regular exercise does help with sleep, but some may find that high-intensity workouts in the evening make them overstimulated when they should be winding down for the night. Aim to keep the really sweaty kind for daytime.*

# So what do we do?

The good news is the principles of balancing blood sugar are incredibly easy to follow, the results are very powerful and, best of all, the effects are immediate. When does *that* ever happen in life?

## SUGAR IS MEAN

Minimise sugary foods otherwise a sugar-happy spike will be followed by a crash and a charming quota of exhaustion and moodiness. Avoid:

▶ *Sweets, fizzy drinks, fruit juice, white bread, pasta, rice, pastries, biscuits, soft tropical fruit like bananas and mangoes.*

## SHOW ME THE FIBRE

The source of carbohydrate is key. The best kind are complex carbohydrates, which are high in fibre for a slow, steady release of energy:

▶ *Non-starchy veg (broccoli, cauliflower, cabbage, spinach, cucumber, carrots).*
▶ *Starchy vegetables (sweet potatoes, potatoes, peas, butternut squash, corn, parsnips).*
▶ *High-fibre fruit (apples, kiwis, blueberries, raspberries, blackberries, pineapple).*
▶ *Wholegrains (quinoa, rye, millet, oats).*

 *The more you have to chew a vegetable, fruit or grain, the better it is, as it indicates higher levels of beneficial fibre.*

 *Freezing protein-rich foods like fish, poultry or vegan burgers is so easy and super convenient for when you're feeling lazy.*

## THE MANY FACES OF FRUIT

Fruit is a mixed bag. Most of it is packed with antioxidants and plant chemicals, both of which are highly beneficial. Some fruits are fibre-rich, but many can also be pretty sugary. The best way to judge its credentials is on the glycaemic index. As a general rule, the less sweet and more it needs to be chewed, the better:

▶ *Green apples, kiwis, citrus (oranges, grapefruit), berries (blueberries, raspberries, blackberries, strawberries), peaches, plums, pears, pomegranate seeds.*

## THE POWER OF PROTEIN

It is essential to combine carbohydrates with protein to slow down the release of sugar into the bloodstream and keep levels stable:

▶ *Animal sources: lean meat (chicken, turkey, red meat), fish (salmon, mackerel, cod, sea bass, haddock, tuna), shellfish (prawns, mussels, clams, oysters, crab, crayfish), dairy products (milk, yogurt, kefir), eggs.*
▶ *Plant sources: nuts (almonds, cashews, walnuts, peanuts), seeds (pumpkin, hemp, flax, chia), lentils, chickpeas, beans.*

## SNACKING IS EVERYTHING

People often think snacking refers to a mid-morning biscuit or a packet of crisps. That's obviously not my interpretation. I am a big snack advocate, as something small and healthy can help balance energy levels throughout the day, bridging the gap between meals. The key is using the same GP principles – always including protein and a high-fibre carbohydrate. Any combination of the below will stop the urge to reach for a coffee or something sweet. A proper snack mid-afternoon also decreases the likelihood of overeating at night.

| PROTEIN | CARBOHYDRATE |
|---|---|
| Hard-boiled egg | Oatcakes |
| Hummus, cottage cheese, bean paste | Raw vegetable sticks |
| Nut butter (cashew, almond, hazelnut, peanut) | Fresh or dried fruit (no added sugar) |
| Natural live yogurt or nut yogurt (coconut, almond) | Rye or pumpernickel bread |
| Poultry slices, lean ham, smoked salmon | Crackers (lentil, quinoa, buckwheat, brown rice, chickpea) |

*Aim to eat every 3–4 hours. Never wait until you feel starving, as that indicates your blood sugar has dropped too low. Instead, keep an eye out for signs of peckishness. That's the moment to strike.*

*Seaweed is full of thyroid-supporting iodine and comes in various forms, which can be added to soups, shredded into salads and rice bowls, or eaten as a crunchy toasted snack (like non-evil crisps).*

## EXERCISE = ENERGY

The thought of exercising when the body feels tired sounds like the worst idea anyone ever had. However, some gentle, low-intensity physical activity such as walking, swimming, cycling, yoga and Pilates has been shown to increase energy, rather than get rid of the last remnants of it. This happens through the release of certain hormones. Endorphins, serotonin and dopamine lift the spirits and makes us want to move, while a small release of the stress hormones actually has an energising effect. Exercise can also help the body sleep better at night, which will inevitably have a positive impact on energy levels during the day as they start to rebalance.

*Ditch the energy drinks for vitamin B complex. While it's important to include these in the diet, concentrated supplements will give you the energy of a sugar-charged 3-year-old – just make sure they're always taken with food.*

## THE ENERGISERS
### B vitamins

B vitamins not only help support metabolism, they also play a crucial role in the Krebs cycle. It's not uncommon for people to be deficient in B vitamins and low levels can cause fatigue:

▸ *Animal foods: eggs, fish (salmon, mackerel, tuna), shellfish (prawns, oysters, clams), dairy.*
▸ *Plant foods: leafy green vegetables (spinach, kale, spring greens, Swiss chard), beans (kidney beans, black beans, chickpeas), wholegrain (rye, brown rice, buckwheat).*

### Iron

Iron is an essential component of red blood cells. When iron levels are depleted, production is slowed and cells are deprived of the oxygen needed to process glucose. Without it, they cannot produce the ATP they need for energy – and to survive:

▸ *Animal foods: lean red meat (beef, lamb, pork), seafood (clams, oysters, octopus, mussels, scallops).*
▸ *Plant foods: beans (soya, kidney, lima, black, chickpeas), leafy greens (spinach, Swiss chard, kale), nuts (almonds, cashews, hazelnuts, walnuts, peanuts), seeds (pumpkin, hemp, sesame), mushrooms (button, morels), grains (quinoa, oats, barley).*

### Iodine

Iodine is a key player in the synthesis of thyroid hormones, which help regulate metabolism and the production of energy. Iodine also supports healthy cognitive function, assisting the brain's ability to focus:

▸ *Fish, seaweed (kelp, nori, wakame), shellfish, dairy products, eggs.*

### Ashwagandha

Used for thousands of years across Asia to treat insomnia and fatigue, this herb increases and supports energy levels, stabilises blood sugar and naturally helps to combat stress.

### Red, purple and blue superfoods

Richly coloured superfoods are full of nutrients, including vitamins A and C, iron, zinc and magnesium, which all help maintain energy levels. They also contain high amounts of antioxidants that fight free radicals:

▸ *Blueberries, blackberries, raspberries, strawberries, bilberries, acai berries, cherries, beetroot, aronia berry, goji berries.*

*It's harder to get a good supply of iron in vegetarian diets, whatever Popeye said (liar), so do supplement.*

## Superhero supplements

- Vitamin B complex
- Red/purple/blue superfood powder – individual or combined
- Iron
- Magnesium
- Green tea extract
- Adaptogens – ashwagandha, maca, rhodiola, moringa, reishi
- CoQ10

# 11/
## eat

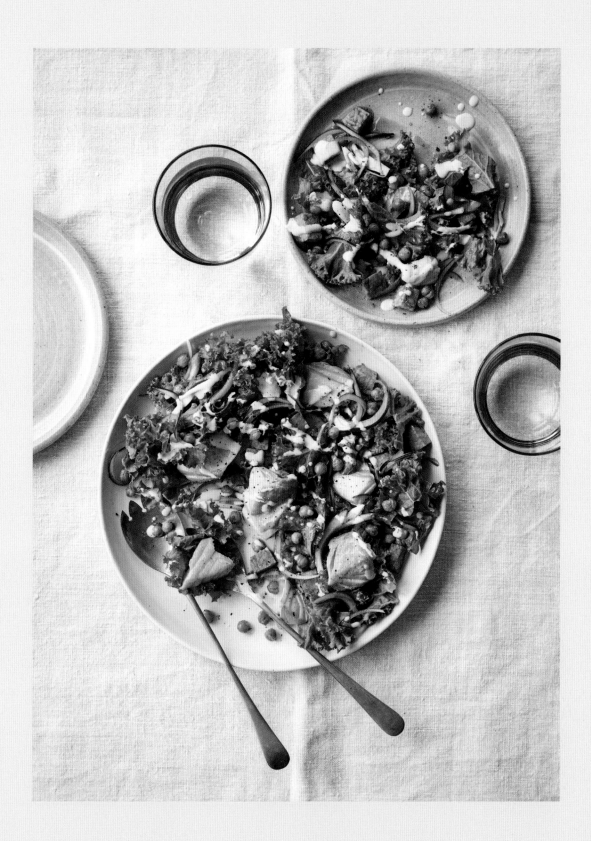

*if using gluten-free oats*

*if using nut yoghurt*

gluten free

dairy free

vegan

# rhubarb & red berry pots

*serves 4*

350g (12oz) rhubarb, chopped into small pieces

3 tablespoons agave syrup

juice of 1½ lemons

1 tablespoon water

40g (1½oz) rolled oats (gluten free, if preferred)

a small handful of your favourite nuts (about 20g/½oz), chopped

400g (14oz) live Greek or nut yogurt (coconut, almond or cashew)

a handful of red berries (raspberries or strawberries)

Rhubarb is packed with soluble fibre, which is essential for healthy digestion, as well as vitamin K and calcium. This recipe has been designed to be on the tart, refreshing side, so do add a little more agave if you prefer it sweeter. These pots make a great breakfast and can also work as a healthy pudding on mindful days. They will keep in the refrigerator for 4 days, while the toasted nuts will last happily in an airtight container for up to a week.

Preheat the oven to 200°C (400°F), gas mark 6. Arrange the rhubarb in the bottom of a baking dish, making sure the dish is big enough to fit it in a single layer. Add 2 tablespoons of the agave syrup and the lemon juice. Cover the dish tightly with foil.

Mix the rest of the agave syrup with 1 tablespoon of water. Spread the oats and nuts out on a baking tray and coat them with the agave-water mix. Put them both into the oven at the same time. Take the nuts and oats out after about 15 minutes, or when they are lightly golden. Take the rhubarb out about 5 minutes later (it should cook for a total of 20 minutes) or when it is lovely and soft. Leave them both to cool.

Spoon the rhubarb and yogurt in alternate layers into 4 small glasses or pots. Keep in the refrigerator until needed. When ready to eat, sprinkle over the toasted oats and nuts and the red berries.

| PREP 5 minutes | COOK 20 minutes | CALORIES<br>170 with coconut yogurt<br>163 with almond yogurt |
| --- | --- | --- |

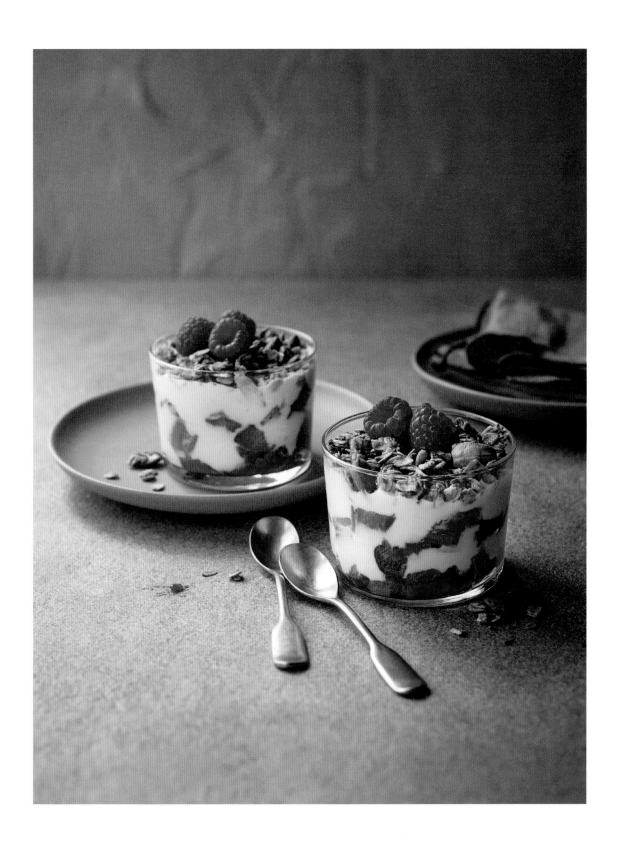

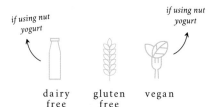

if using nut
yogurt

if using nut
yogurt

dairy
free

gluten
free

vegan

# chia & berries
# overnight bowl

*serves 2*

85g (3oz) raspberries
100g (3½oz) natural live or nut
  yogurt
200ml (7fl oz) almond milk
4 tablespoons chia seeds
1 tablespoon agave syrup
a squeeze of lemon juice

*to serve*
a handful of mixed berries
pinch of lemon zest

Chia seeds are high in protein, fibre and omega-3, which has many health benefits, from reducing inflammation to improving skin health and hormone balance. Soaking the seeds overnight makes them easier to digest, allowing their nutrients to be absorbed more effectively. Swirl the raspberries through for a vivid-red antioxidant boost.

Place the raspberries in a jar or container with a lid and break them up using a fork. Add the yogurt, milk, chia seeds, agave and lemon juice and mix well. Cover with the lid and refrigerate overnight or for a minimum of 6 hours.

Serve in a bowl with a handful of berries and finish with the lemon zest.

| PREP 5 minutes | CHILL 6 hours or overnight | CALORIES 218 with plain live yogurt 204 with almond yogurt |
|---|---|---|

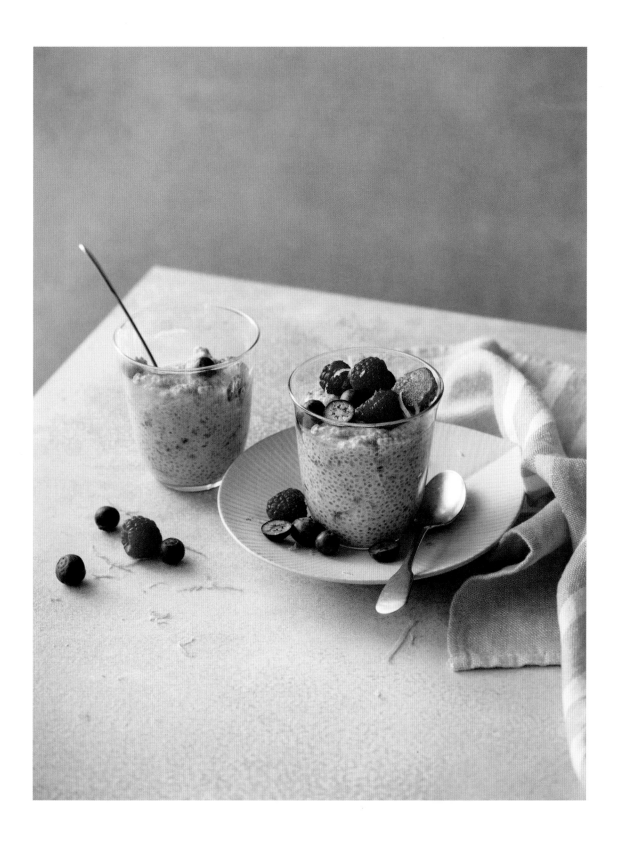

# vegan breakfast bars

*if using gluten-free oats*

dairy free    gluten free    vegan

*makes 10 bars*

60g (2¼oz) cashew butter

2 tablespoons agave syrup

150g (5½oz) Medjool dates, pitted and roughly chopped

4 tablespoons pumpkin seeds

4 tablespoons chia seeds

100g (3½oz) jumbo rolled oats (gluten free, if preferred)

50g (1¾oz) almonds, chopped

These super-convenient bars are packed with protein and make a great breakfast on- the- go or a delicious mid-afternoon snack. They will live happily in the refrigerator for up to 3 days in an airtight container and in the freezer for up to 1 month – just remember to take them out to thaw in advance.

Line a 20cm (8 inch) square baking tin with non-stick baking paper. Melt the nut butter and agave in a small saucepan over a low heat.

Meanwhile, blitz the dates in a food processor until they come together in a soft ball. If they're not looking sticky enough, add a tablespoon of boiling water and blitz again.

In a large bowl, mix the date paste with all the remaining ingredients and add the melted nut butter and agave. With clean hands, get stuck in and mix everything together, until all the ingredients have been evenly dispersed.

Spoon the mixture into the lined tin and smooth over the top. Cover and chill in the fridge for 20 minutes until firm to the touch, then cut into 10 bars.

| PREP 10 minutes | CHILL 20 minutes | CALORIES 213 p/bar |
| --- | --- | --- |

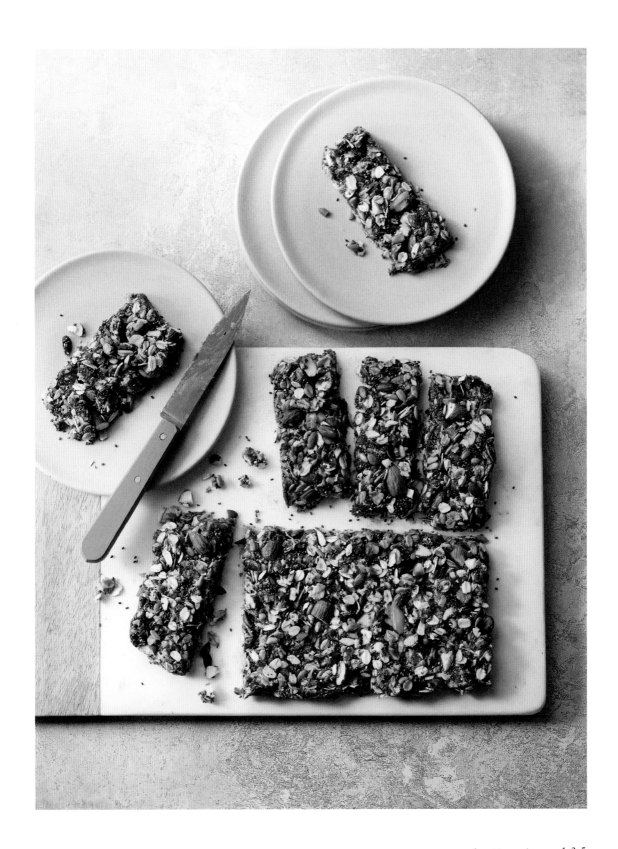

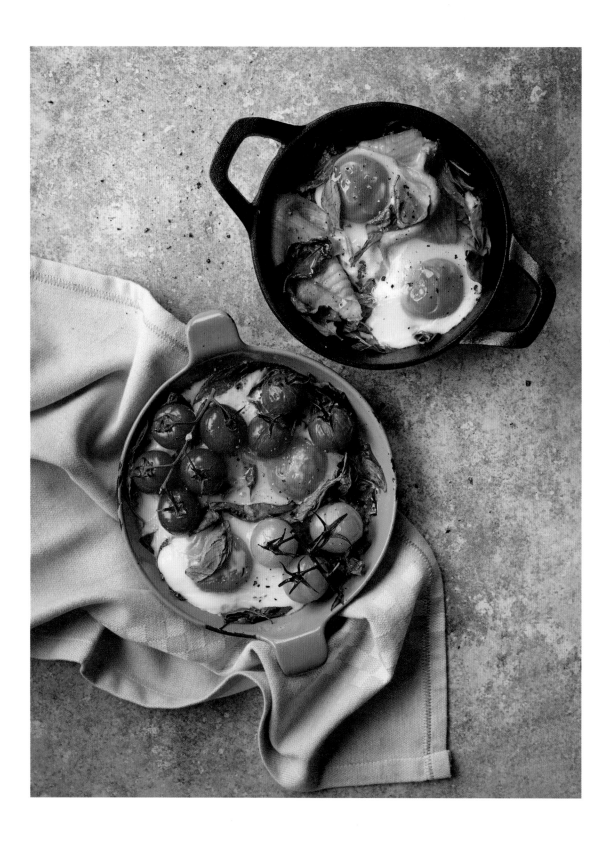

# anytime
# baked eggs

dairy
free

gluten
free

It is joyful how quick and simple this recipe is. Not only does it work brilliantly as a shared brunch, it is particularly good for any lurking hangovers, as smoked salmon is one of the best sources of omega-3 and will help the liver to cleanse the body of the remnants of last night's revelry. As for tomato and basil, it's one of my all-time favourite combinations. Fresh, clean and so easy, this dish practically makes itself.

Preheat the oven to 220°C (425°F), gas mark 7. Lightly grease 2 small ovenproof dishes with the oil.

Line one with the spinach and smoked salmon. Line the other with the tomatoes and basil. Crack two eggs over each filling and season. Bake for 8–10 minutes, or until the whites have set and the yolks are still oozy.

*serves 2*

1 teaspoon olive oil

a small handful of spinach (about 40g/1½oz), chopped

80g (3oz) smoked salmon

100g (3½oz) cherry tomatoes, chopped

a small handful of basil (about 15g/½oz)

4 large organic or free-range eggs

sea salt and freshly ground black pepper

| PREP 5 minutes | COOK 10 minutes | CALORIES 267 |
| --- | --- | --- |

*if using nut yogurt and dairy-free chocolate*

*if using gluten-free oats*

*if using nut yogurt and vegan chocolate*

dairy
free

gluten
free

vegan

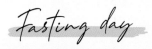
*Fasting day*

# chocolate breakfast oats

What's not to love? This is hassle-free (all the magic happens overnight) and feels like a treat because – hello – chocolate for breakfast! Permission is given to add some dark chocolate shavings (I'm in a generous mood today). This will keep in the fridge in an airtight container for 4 days.

*serves 1*

100g (3½oz) natural live yogurt or nut yogurt

4 tablespoons coconut milk

1 tablespoon unsweetened cacao powder

2 teaspoons agave syrup

20g (¾oz) rolled oats

a sprinkle of dark chocolate shavings (optional), to serve

Place all the ingredients except the chocolate shavings in a jar or container with a lid and stir so that everything is mixed well. Put the lid on and refrigerate overnight or for a minimum of 8 hours. To serve, sprinkle over the chocolate.

| PREP 5 minutes | CHILL 8 hours or overnight | CALORIES 247 with plain live yogurt 288 with coconut yogurt |
|---|---|---|

gluten
free

veggie

# speedy veggie omelette

Using yogurt and only one egg makes this lighter than a normal omelette, without compromising on protein. I like adding mushrooms and spinach, but any vegetables will work if softened first. It makes a lovely cooked breakfast but would also work as a light lunch or supper.

*serves 1*

1½ teaspoons rapeseed oil

1 garlic clove, grated

30g (1oz) mushrooms (button, chestnut or wild), thinly sliced

80g (3oz) spinach, chopped

1 large egg

1 large tablespoon natural live or almond yogurt

sea salt and black pepper

a small handful of chives (about 15g/½oz), finely chopped, to serve

Heat the oil in a frying pan over a medium heat and gently sauté the garlic and mushrooms for 2–3 minutes, or until the mushrooms start to pick up a little colour. Add the spinach and let it wilt. A tiny splash of water will help, if needed.

In a bowl, whisk the egg, stir in the yogurt and pour into the pan. Cook for a minute or two. Serve with the chives.

| PREP 5 minutes | COOK 5 minutes | CALORIES 172 with plain live yogurt 168 with almond yogurt |
|---|---|---|

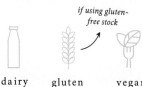

*if using gluten-free stock*

dairy free   gluten free   vegan

# green superfood soup

*serves 2*

1 tablespoon rapeseed or coconut oil

3 garlic cloves, grated

2cm (1 inch) piece of fresh ginger, peeled and grated

½ teaspoon ground turmeric

150g (5½oz) courgettes, chopped

750ml (1⅓ pint) vegetable stock (fresh, bouillon or cubes are fine)

120g (4½oz) kale, stalks removed

100g (3½oz) broccoli, cut into small florets

4 tablespoons lemon juice

a handful of parsley (about 15g/½oz), chopped

sea salt and freshly ground black pepper

This alkalising green soup is ideal for fasting days because of the high fibre content of the cruciferous vegetables. Spiced with the anti-inflammatory ginger and turmeric, this is the recipe I turn to when I feel like my liver needs a bit of attention.

Heat the oil in a saucepan over a medium heat. Add the garlic, ginger and turmeric, stirring for a couple of minutes until fragrant.

Add the courgettes and cook for 3 minutes, ensuring they're well coated with the spice mix, then add half the stock and let it simmer away for 3 minutes.

Add the kale, broccoli, lemon juice and the remaining stock, cooking for a further 3 minutes, or until the vegetables feel soft when prodded with the tip of a knife.

Remove from the heat and add most of the parsley before pouring it all into a blender. Blitz until velvety smooth and season to taste. Serve with the remaining parsley sprinkled over the top.

| PREP 10 minutes | COOK 15 minutes | CALORIES 141 |
|---|---|---|

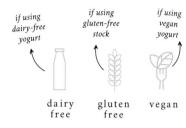

# turmeric-infused lentil & carrot soup

if using
dairy-free
yogurt

if using
gluten-free
stock

if using
vegan
yogurt

dairy
free

gluten
free

vegan

*serves 4*

1 tablespoon olive oil

1 red onion, chopped

4 large carrots, chopped

1 teaspoon ground turmeric

1 teaspoon ground cumin

1 litre (1¾ pints) vegetable stock
  (fresh, bouillon or cubes are fine)

5 tablespoons Puy lentils (about
  70g/2½oz)

4 tablespoons natural live yogurt
  (or almond as a vegan alternative)

sea salt and freshly ground
  black pepper

*to serve*

pinch of chilli flakes

a small handful of fresh coriander
  or parsley (about 15g/½oz),
  finely chopped

Turmeric is an anti-inflammatory wonder nutrient that's both aromatic and delicious. The lentils are high in protein and fibre, which makes this soup satisfying and filling but still reassuringly low in calories.

Heat the oil in a large saucepan over a medium heat. Add the onion and carrots and cook for 10 minutes until softened.

Add the turmeric and cumin and fry for a minute until fragrant, then add the vegetable stock and the lentils. Bring to the boil, then reduce the heat and simmer for 20 minutes until the lentils are cooked through.

Pour into a blender and blitz until silky and smooth, then return the soup to the pan and heat until piping hot. Season to taste with salt and pepper.

Divide between 4 bowls and finish with a dollop of yogurt, some chilli flakes and a sprinkling of herbs.

| PREP 5 minutes | COOK 35 minutes | CALORIES<br>142 with plain live yogurt<br>138 with almond yogurt |
| --- | --- | --- |

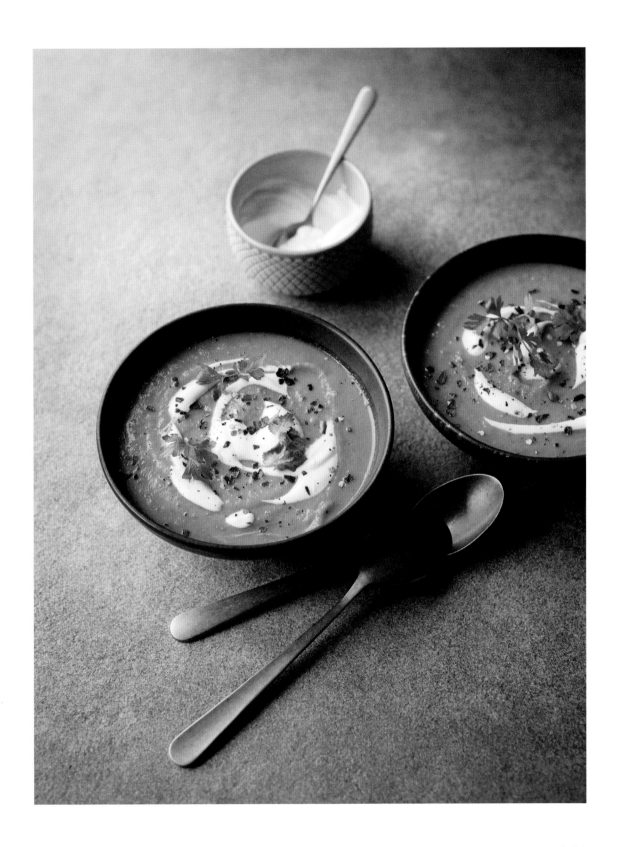

# chorizo & edamame salad with a poached egg

check the chorizo
is gluten free

dairy
free

gluten
free

*serves* 2

80g (3oz) frozen edamame
(soya) beans

50g (1¾oz) cooking chorizo,
cut into cubes

1 shallot, finely chopped

1 teaspoon rapeseed oil (only
if needed)

100g (3½oz) rocket

juice of 1 small lemon

2 organic or free-range eggs,
cooked to preference

sea salt and freshly ground
black pepper

Chorizo in small amounts is fine on a fasting day, adding a hearty helping of flavour and plenty of spice. Edamame is a great combination of protein and fibre, both of which are perfect for weight loss because they help us to feel fuller for longer and ward off cravings. Feel free to cook the egg to preference – I happen to love mine poached.

Add the edamame to a pan of salted boiling water and cook for 3½ minutes, when they should be al dente. Remove from the heat, drain and run them under cold water. Pop them out of their pods if they are whole. Set aside in a bowl.

In a frying pan over a medium heat, fry the chorizo for 8–10 minutes. Add the shallot and fry for a further 5 minutes, only adding the rapeseed oil if needed (chorizo can produce a bit of oil, so it may not be necessary to add more). Add to the bowl with the edamame beans, along with the rocket and lemon juice, mix everything together, then season to taste.

Divide between 2 plates, top each with an egg and serve.

| PREP 5 minutes | COOK 25 minutes | CALORIES 226 |
|---|---|---|

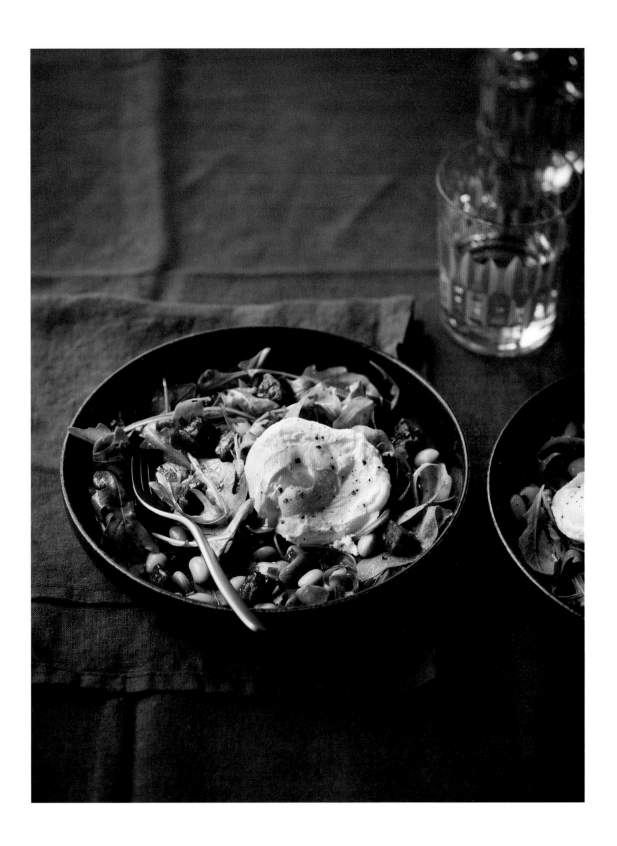

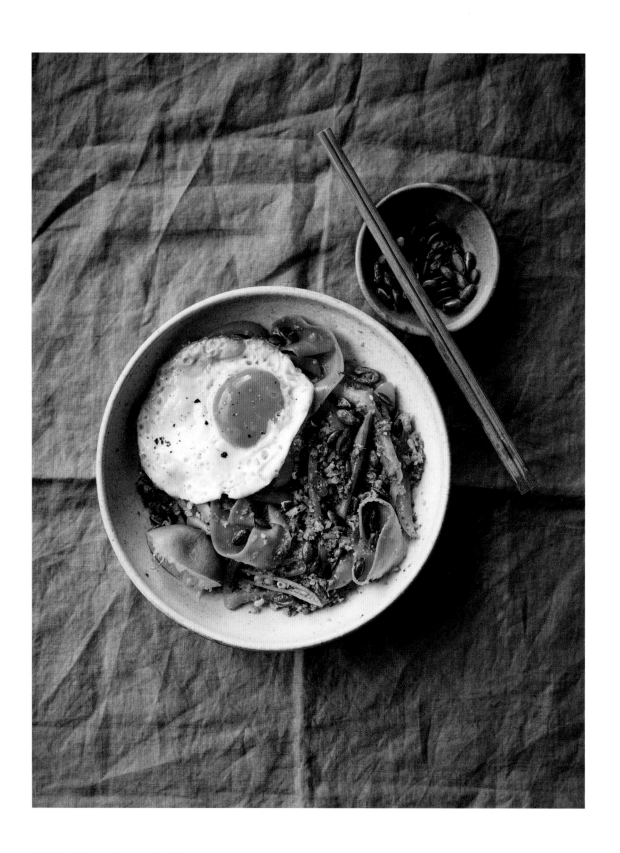

# green fried rice

*if using tamari*

gluten   veggie
free

Broccoli rice is a high-fibre alternative to its distant cousin. Cruciferous vegetables are packed with immunity-supporting antioxidants, and adding an egg on top gives it that extra dose of protein. This dish has a touch of Thai thrown into the mix... always a joy.

Place the chopped broccoli stalk in a food processor and blitz it thoroughly until it looks like grains of rice. Transfer to a bowl. Blitz the florets, then add them to the same bowl.

Next, blitz the ginger, garlic and onion in the food processor.

Heat the sesame oil in a frying pan over a medium heat, then gently fry the ginger, garlic and onion mixture for a couple of minutes, or until fragrant. Then add the broccoli rice, along with two tablespoons of water, the yellow pepper and most of the chilli, and fry for about 5 minutes. The broccoli should start to take on a bit of colour at this point. Throw in the carrot and sugar snap peas.

In a small bowl, mix the sugar, tamari or soy, tamarind paste and most of the lime juice before adding it to the pan. Season with salt and pepper. Make sure everything is nicely coated with the sauce and fry for a further 5 minutes.

Divide between 2 plates and season well. Serve each topped with an egg, cooked the way you like it best, along with the seeds, the rest of the chilli and a squeeze of lime.

*serves* 2

1 small head of broccoli (about 300g/10½oz), cut into florets and stalk trimmed and roughly chopped

2cm (1 inch) piece of fresh ginger, peeled and grated

2 garlic cloves, grated

1 onion, chopped

1 teaspoon toasted sesame oil

2 tablespoons water

1 yellow pepper, cored, deseeded and thinly sliced

1 red chilli, deseeded and thinly sliced

1 carrot, thinly sliced or spiralised

a handful of sugar snap peas (about 20g/½oz)

1 teaspoon coconut sugar

2 tablespoons tamari or soy sauce

2 tablespoons tamarind paste

juice of 1 lime

2 eggs, cooked to preference

sea salt and freshly ground black pepper

1 tablespoon pumpkin seeds, to serve

| PREP 10 minutes | COOK 25 minutes | CALORIES 242 |
|---|---|---|

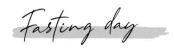

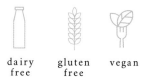

dairy
free

gluten
free

vegan

# cauliflower steaks with olive & caper salsa

serves 2

1 large cauliflower

1 teaspoon olive oil

pinch of paprika

2 tablespoons flaked almonds

1 teaspoon vegan butter

2 tablespoons pitted green olives,
  chopped

1 teaspoon capers, drained

2 tablespoons apple cider vinegar

a small handful of parsley, chopped

sea salt and freshly ground
  black pepper

Cauliflower steaks are all the rage at the moment and rightly so, as cruciferous vegetables are very good at supporting healthy liver function. They are roasted in the oven here, but try them on the barbecue in summer as a vegan option. Serve with a handful of rocket spritzed in lemon juice as a cheerful little sidekick.

Preheat the oven to 200°C (400°F), gas mark 6 and line a baking tray with non-stick baking paper.

Trim a little off the stalk of the cauliflower before carefully cutting 2 slices (roughly 2cm/¾ inch thick) through the middle (the stalk will hold them together). Save the rest to make soup or cauliflower rice.

Lightly brush each side of the steaks with the oil. Season with salt, pepper and paprika, then roast for 20–25 minutes, carefully turning them over halfway through the cooking time, until they start to turn a light golden brown and feel tender when prodded with a fork.

Lightly toast the almond flakes in a hot, dry frying pan over a medium heat for a few minutes, keeping an eye on them to make sure they don't catch. Melt the butter in a saucepan over a medium heat, then toss in the chopped olives and capers and cook for about 2 minutes until they start to slightly crisp up. Switch off the heat and stir in the apple cider vinegar and parsley. Drizzle the salsa over the steaks and scatter over the almonds to serve.

| PREP 5 minutes | COOK 35 minutes | CALORIES 227 |
| --- | --- | --- |

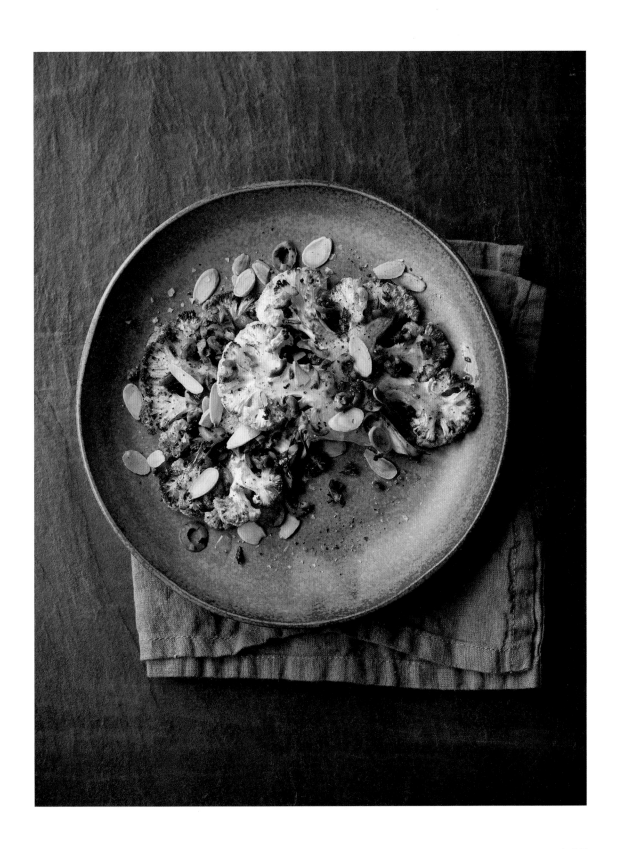

*if using
tamari*

dairy
free

gluten
free

# salmon & ginger
# fishcake bites

*serves* 2 (makes 6 bites)

2 skinless salmon fillets (about
  130g/4½oz each), roughly
  chopped

2cm (1 inch) piece of fresh
  ginger, peeled

1 garlic clove

½ red chili, deseeded and
  roughly chopped

a small handful of chives (about
  10g/¼oz), roughly chopped

½ tablespoon mixed seeds
  (pumpkin and sunflower)

1 teaspoon tamari or soy sauce

1 tablespoon rapeseed oil

juice of 1 lime

Omega-3 reigns supreme in these little Asian-inspired
fishcakes, thanks to the salmon and seed combination.
Eat them piping hot out of the pan and serve with salad or
steamed greens as a light lunch or supper, or make them in
advance – they're just as delicious cold.

Put the salmon, ginger, garlic, chili, chives, seeds and soy or
tamari into a food processor and pulse until blended but still
with a bit of texture.

Tip the mixture out and form into 6 small fishcakes, pressing
them down a little to flatten. Cover and chill in the fridge for
10 minutes.

Heat the oil in a large frying pan over a medium heat and
fry the fishcakes for about 3 minutes on each side, or until
cooked through. Squeeze over the lime juice and serve.

| PREP 10 minutes | CHILL 10 minutes<br>COOK 10 minutes | CALORIES 297 |
|---|---|---|

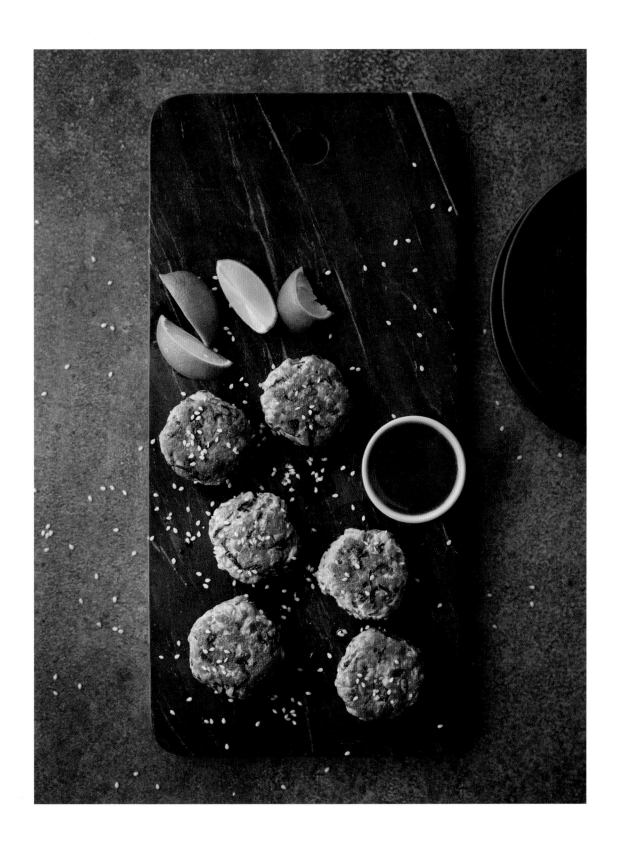

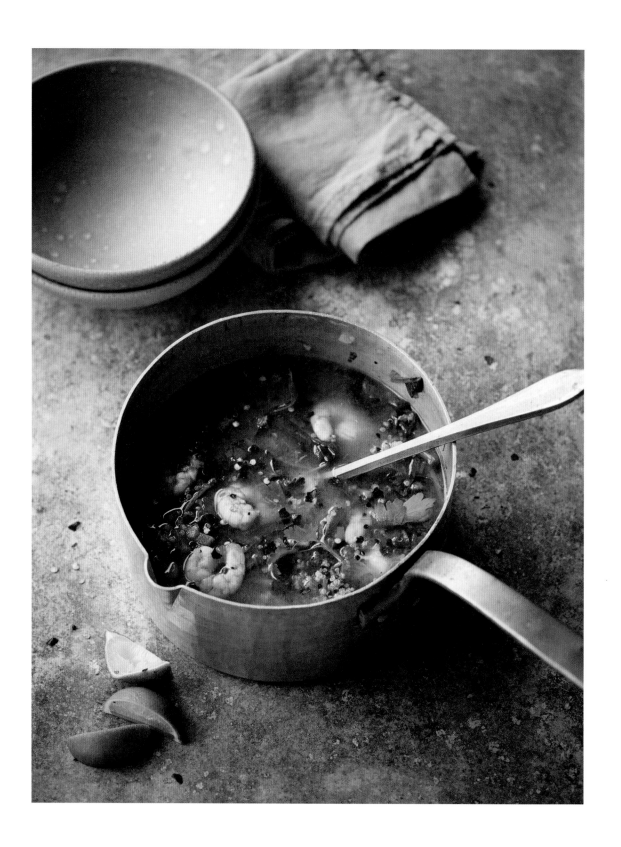

# light vegetable broth with prawns & quinoa

*if using gluten-free stock*

dairy free    gluten free

Fasting days can sound a bit ominous, but this protein-rich soup is surprisingly filling, yet it has the major bonus of being low in calories. The prawns and quinoa combined with the high-fibre vegetables will help balance blood sugar levels throughout the day, preventing energy dips.

Heat the oil in a saucepan over a medium heat and fry the onion for 5 minutes, or until softened.

Add the garlic, quinoa and carrots and fry for a further 5 minutes, stirring constantly. Add the stock, bring to the boil, then reduce the heat and simmer for 15 minutes. By this point, the quinoa should be cooked through.

Stir in the prawns and spinach, simmering for a further couple of minutes until the prawns have turned pale pink. Take off the heat, stir in the lime juice (and zest, if using) and most of the parsley, season to taste and serve with the remaining parsley sprinkled over the top with a pinch of chilli flakes or cayenne pepper.

*serves 2*

1 teaspoon rapeseed oil (or coconut oil)

1 small onion, finely chopped

3 garlic cloves, grated

30g (1¼oz) precooked quinoa

2 small carrots, finely chopped

1 litre (1¾ pints) vegetable stock (fresh, bouillon or cubes are fine)

150g (5½oz) raw peeled king prawns

120g (4½oz) spinach, chopped

juice of 1 lime (add a little of the zest, if you like)

a small handful of parsley (about 15g/½oz), roughly chopped

sea salt and freshly ground black pepper

pinch of chilli flakes or cayenne pepper, to serve

| PREP 5 minutes | COOK 30 minutes | CALORIES 157 |
|---|---|---|

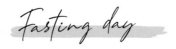

dairy
free

gluten
free

# greens, eggs & ham salad

*serves* 2

2 organic or free-range eggs,
   at room temperature
100g (3½oz) green beans,
   topped and tailed
150g (5½oz) salad leaves
6 cherry tomatoes, halved
¼ small red onion, thinly sliced
80g (3½oz) cooked ham hock,
   shredded
sea salt and freshly ground
   black pepper

*for the dressing*

1 tablespoon extra virgin olive oil
2 teaspoons apple cider vinegar
1 teaspoon Dijon mustard
1 teaspoon agave syrup, to taste

If you're craving a ham sandwich during periods of fasting, this recipe might hit the spot. I'm not in the business of telling people to cut out all the things that they love, so adding ham to a salad is a great alternative to a more calorific sandwich.

To keep the cooking time down (and reduce the washing-up), cook the eggs and beans in the same pan. Add the eggs to a saucepan of boiling water. After 4 minutes, add the beans and cook for a further 3 minutes. Remove both the eggs and the beans (the eggs will have boiled for a total of 7 minutes), drain and run them under cold water until cooled. Peel the eggs and cut them into quarters.

Mix the dressing ingredients together in a small bowl or jug and season. Put the salad leaves, cherry tomatoes, onion and ham into a salad bowl, pour over the dressing and mix well. Place the eggs on top and serve.

| PREP 5 minutes | COOK 10 minutes | CALORIES 233 |
| --- | --- | --- |

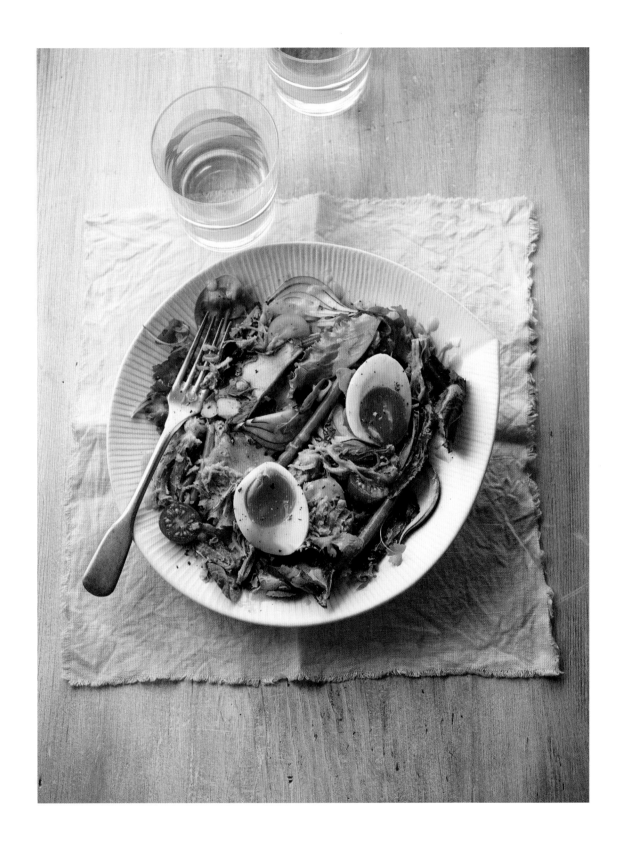

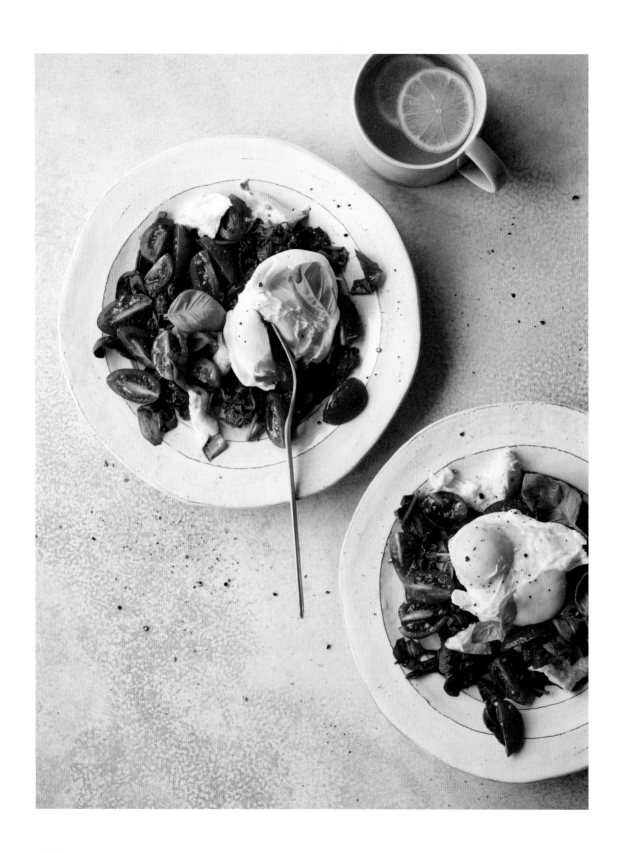

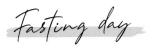 

# tricolore eggs

gluten
free

veggie

The Mediterranean diet is fantastically healthy for the heart and cardiovascular system, as it's based on the simple, fresh ingredients traditionally used throughout Italy, Greece and Spain. This quick recipe is so easy to throw together – the eggs and mozzarella provide the protein element, while the tomatoes, basil and spinach are packed with phytonutrients.

*serves 2*

a squeeze of lemon juice

2 eggs

3 large handfuls of spinach (about 220g/8oz), chopped

10 cherry tomatoes, quartered

50g (1¾oz) mozzarella, torn

1 handful of fresh basil (about 15g/½oz), torn

2 teaspoons extra virgin olive oil

1 teaspoon apple cider vinegar

sea salt and freshly ground black pepper

Heat a saucepan of water over a medium heat until gently simmering, then add a squeeze of lemon juice and crack in the eggs. Poach for 4 minutes.

While the eggs are cooking, place the spinach in a saucepan over a medium heat, add a splash of water and let it wilt. Drain, squeezing out as much of the excess water as possible, and divide between 2 plates.

Mix the tomatoes, mozzarella and basil together in a bowl and coat with the oil and vinegar. Season and mix everything together again well. Spoon on top of the spinach.

Serve each plate with a poached egg on top.

| PREP 8 minutes | COOK 5 minutes | CALORIES 204 |
| --- | --- | --- |

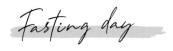

*Fasting day*

dairy
free

gluten
free

# spring greens, chicken & lentil soup

*serves 2*

2 teaspoons rapeseed oil

½ red onion, finely chopped

3 carrots, finely chopped

2 celery sticks, finely chopped

1 organic or free-range chicken
  breast (about 180g/6oz),
  thinly sliced

500ml (18fl oz) chicken or
  vegetable stock (fresh, bouillon
  or cubes are fine)

100g (3½oz) precooked Puy lentils

130g (4½oz) spring greens, cut
  into thin ribbons

juice of 1 lime

a small handful parsley (about
  15g/½oz), chopped

sea salt and freshly ground
  black pepper

Spring greens are high in vitamin C, which supports immunity, and vitamin K, which builds bone strength. I've used precooked lentils here because they're so much easier and quicker – a bonus on fasting days in particular. In combination with the chicken, lentils are a great source of protein, as well as fibre, which will help you to feel fuller for longer. You could swap out the spring greens for any kind of green vegetable – try cabbage, kale or cavolo nero.

Heat the oil in a saucepan over a medium heat and gently fry the onions for about 3 minutes. Add the carrots and celery and cook for a further 6 minutes until they have all softened.

Next, add the chicken and fry for a couple of minutes until it has a little colour and then pour in the stock. Next add the lentils and gently simmer for 5 minutes, then add the spring greens for a further 5 minutes.

Remove the pan from the heat, add the lime juice and season to taste. Stir in the parsley and serve.

| PREP 10 minutes | COOK 25 minutes | CALORIES 246 |
| --- | --- | --- |

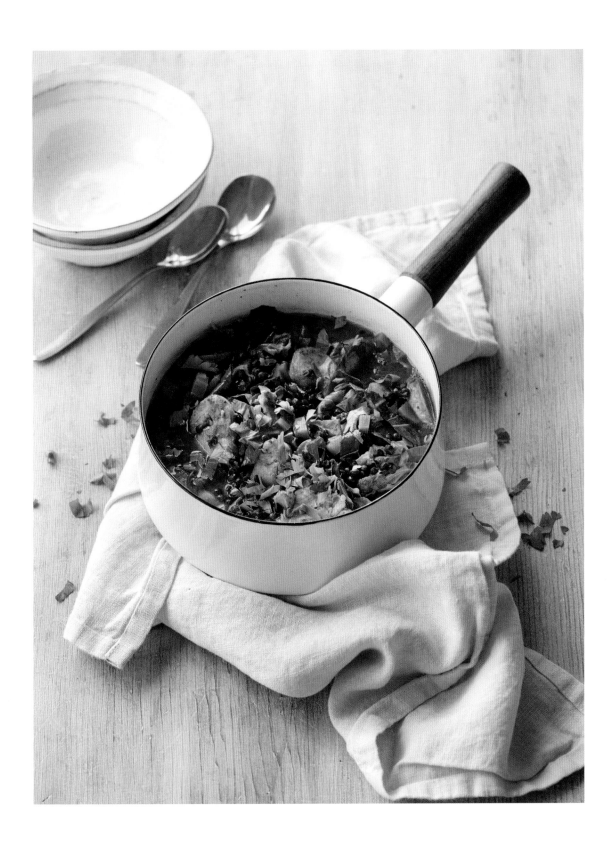

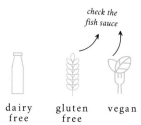

*check the fish sauce*

dairy free    gluten free    vegan

# Thai-spiced vegetable & coconut curry

*serves 2*

½ head of cauliflower (about 180g/6oz), roughly chopped

1 teaspoon olive oil

½ teaspoon ground turmeric

½ teaspoon ground ginger

½ teaspoon sweet paprika

½ teaspoon chilli flakes

300ml (10fl oz) unsweetened coconut milk (also called coconut drink)

120g (4½oz) bean sprouts

120g (4½oz) cabbage, shredded or finely chopped

120g (4½oz) carrots, shredded or finely chopped

1 tablespoon fish sauce

juice of 1 lime

a small handful of basil or Thai basil, if available, (about 15g/½oz), chopped

a small handful of fresh coriander (about 15g/½oz), chopped

100g (3½oz) radishes, thinly sliced

sea salt and freshly ground black pepper

This is a light, fresh alternative to a traditional curry. It is quick to rustle up and makes a deliciously zingy, fragrant lunch or supper for a fasting day. A note about coconut milk: the canned variety is significantly higher in calories, so try to find the kind that is sold in a carton, which is lighter.

Preheat the oven to 200°C (400°F), gas mark 6.

Place the cauliflower in a roasting tin, add the oil and mix together well, then season. Roast for about 20 minutes, turning halfway, until it has softened and turned golden.

Meanwhile, heat a saucepan over a medium heat, add the turmeric, ginger, paprika, chilli flakes and coconut milk, and bring up to a gentle simmer while stirring constantly. Cover with a lid, reduce the heat to low and cook for 5 minutes, when it should start to become fragrant.

Stir in the bean sprouts, cabbage and carrots, and cook for a further 5 minutes, or until tender (but they still have a little bite). Add the fish sauce, lime juice and half the herbs, stirring well. Season to taste.

Serve the cauliflower with the vegetables, radishes and remaining herbs.

| PREP 10 minutes | COOK 20 minutes | CALORIES 193 |
|---|---|---|

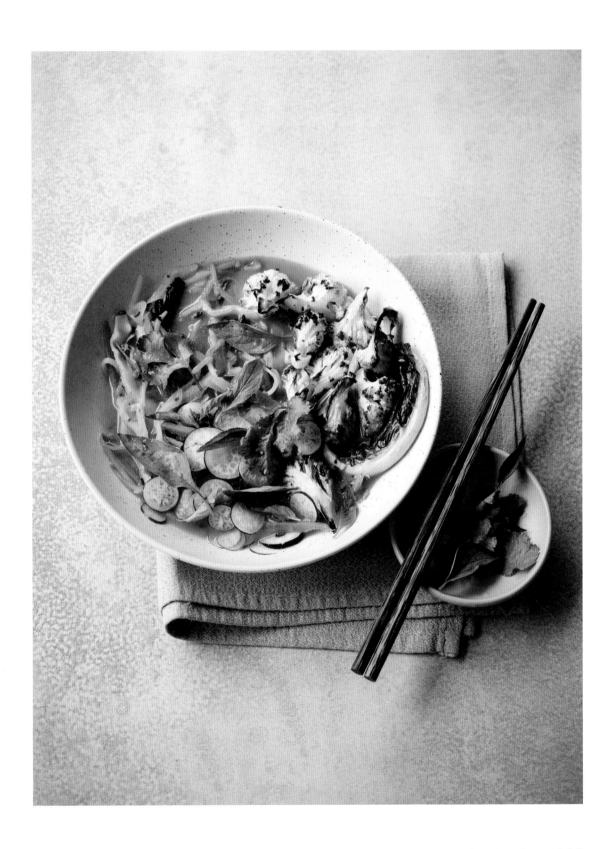

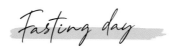

dairy
free

gluten
free

# kimchi salad with turkey & quinoa

*serves* 2

8 mushrooms of your choice
(chestnut, shiitake, button),
thinly sliced

100g (3½oz) radishes, thinly sliced

150g (5½oz) precooked quinoa

150g (5½oz) kimchi

1 tablespoon sesame oil

½ bag mixed salad leaves (about
50g/1¾oz)

a small handful of fresh coriander
(about 15g/½oz), chopped

40g (1½oz) precooked turkey or
chicken breast, sliced

Kimchi is the Korean sauerkraut. It's fermented vegetables with added spices and has health benefits coming out of its ears. Your microbiome will be extremely happy with you if you eat kimchi, as it contains good bacteria created during the fermentation process. Its tangy flavour works well with a light white meat such as turkey or chicken – but stick with the amount of meat suggested to avoid wandering off the calorie target for a fasting day.

Place the mushrooms, radishes, quinoa and kimchi in a bowl, add the sesame oil and mix everything together.

Divide the salad leaves between 2 plates and spoon over the quinoa mix. Sprinkle with the coriander. Finally, add the turkey or chicken, either mixing it in or serving it on the side.

| PREP 5 minutes | CALORIES 213 (with turkey) 219 (with chicken) |
| --- | --- |

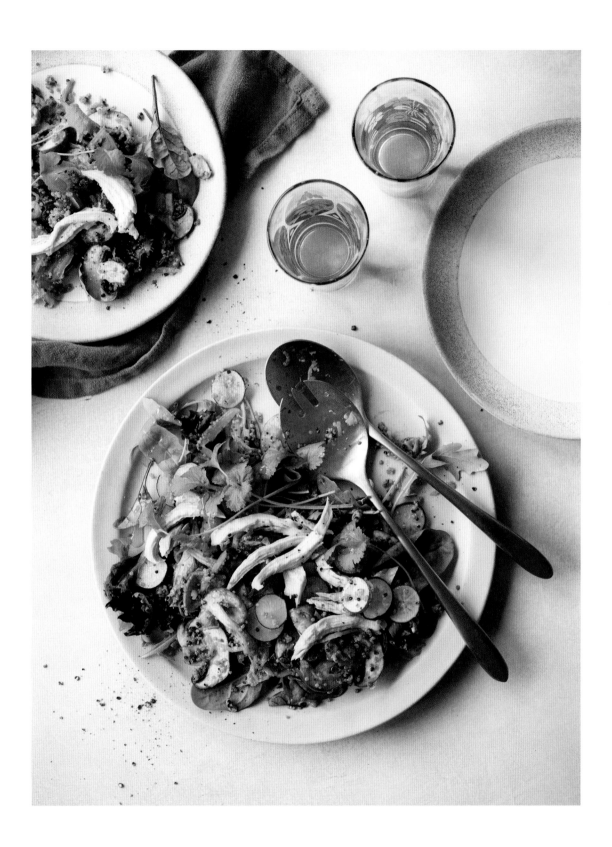

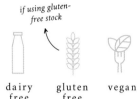

*if using gluten-
free stock*

dairy
free

gluten
free

vegan

# mushroom & lentil bolognese with courgetti

*serves* 2

½ tablespoon rapeseed oil

1 onion, finely chopped

3 garlic cloves, grated

1 small carrot, grated

2 celery sticks, finely chopped

75g (2½oz) mushrooms of your
  choice (chestnut, button),
  thickly sliced

250g (9oz) passata or canned
  chopped tomatoes

500ml (18fl oz) vegetable stock
  (fresh, bouillon or cubes are fine)

250g (9oz) Puy lentils

a small sprig of rosemary

pinch of dried oregano

1 tablespoon apple cider vinegar

1 large courgette, spiralised

sea salt and freshly ground
  black pepper

If you love Italian food as much as I do, this recipe will strike a chord. Lentils (particularly good for heart and digestive health) and mushrooms take the place of minced beef, with courgetti replacing pasta, making a light and delicious alternative to the classic spaghetti Bolognese. The portions may feel a little on the generous side, so any leftover sauce can happily live in the freezer for up to 3 months.

Heat the oil in a large saucepan (preferably one that has a lid) over a medium heat. Add the onion, garlic, carrot and celery and fry for 8 minutes, or until softened.

Add the mushrooms and fry for a further 2 minutes before adding the passata or canned tomatoes, stock, lentils, rosemary, oregano and vinegar.

Cover and leave to simmer for about 20 minutes, stirring occasionally, until the lentils are tender. Remove the rosemary sprig.

Mix in the courgetti (you could briefly flash-fry it in a pan, but the heat of the sauce will warm it through) and season to taste before serving.

| PREP 15 minutes | COOK 35 minutes | CALORIES 279 |
| --- | --- | --- |

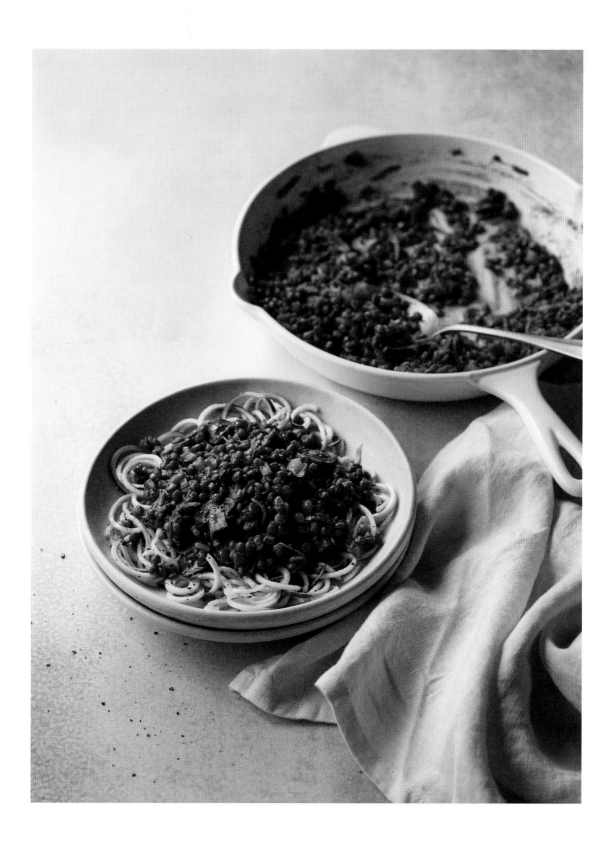

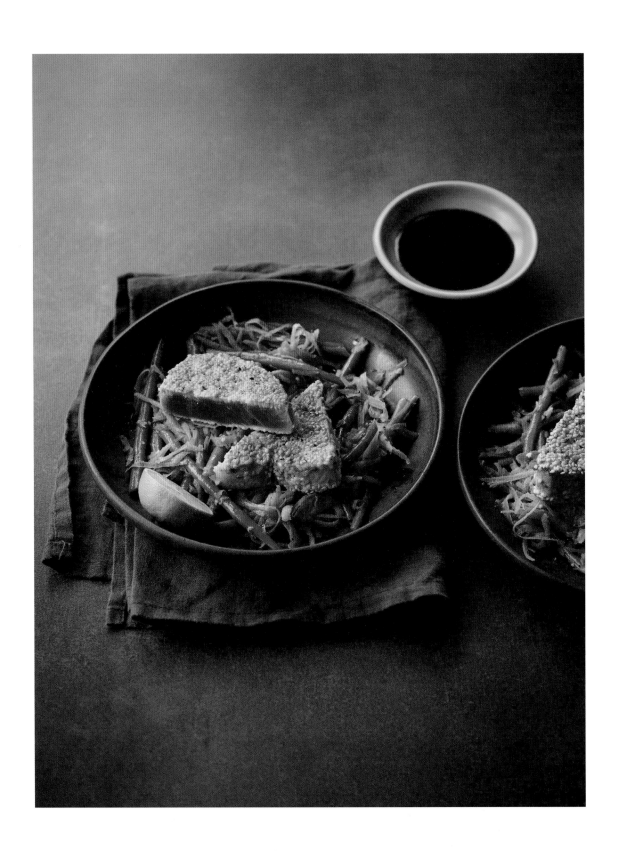

# seared sesame tuna with green beans & carrots

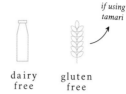

*if using tamari*

dairy
free

gluten
free

Tuna is quite a meaty fish, so it can be a good replacement for red meat, which should be eaten sparingly. It also happens to be very high in selenium, a natural antioxidant and, along with the crunchy sesame seeds, is an excellent source of essential fatty acids.

Season and coat the tuna steak in the sesame seeds, pressing them in gently so they stick.

Heat half the oil in a frying pan over a medium heat and then add the beans, along with a splash of water, and cook for a couple of minutes. Next add the carrots and cook for a further minute before adding the tamari or soy and stirring well. Remove from the heat (the vegetables should still have a bite to them) and transfer to a plate.

Using the same pan, heat the rest of the oil and sear the tuna for a minute or two on each side (this will depend on the thickness of the fish and how rare you like it).

Place the tuna on top of the crunchy vegetables and squeeze over the lime juice before serving.

*serves 1*

1 tuna steak (about 100g/3½oz)

1 teaspoon sesame seeds

1 teaspoon rapeseed oil

120g (4½oz) green beans, topped and tailed

1 small carrot, grated or spiralised

1 teaspoon tamari or soy sauce

juice of ½ lime

sea salt and freshly ground black pepper

| PREP 5 minutes | COOK 10 minutes | CALORIES 238 |
| --- | --- | --- |

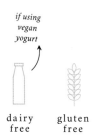

*if using vegan yogurt*

dairy free

gluten free

# steak, kale & asparagus salad

*serves* 2

180g (6oz) fillet steak (or any kind of very lean meat, if preferred)

1 tablespoon rapeseed oil

150g (5½oz) asparagus, woody stalks snapped off

200g (7oz) kale, stalks removed

2 tablespoons natural live yogurt (or almond as a vegan alternative)

juice of ½ lemon

sea salt and freshly ground black pepper

While red meat is not something for every day, it can make an occasional guest appearance – the important thing is always to buy high quality. It's very rich in iron, while asparagus is high in vitamins A, C and K, as well as being low in calories. Kale is so good in so many ways, I could write an entirely separate book on it, if not several volumes.

Heat a griddle pan over a medium-high heat. Cover the steak in the rapeseed oil, season thoroughly and place in the pan, along with the asparagus. Cook the steak for 3 minutes on each side (this will mean it's still quite rare, so cook for longer according to preference) and turn the asparagus occasionally until it gets the tell-tale griddle stripes. Remove from the heat, let the steak rest for 10 minutes and set aside the asparagus on a warmed plate.

While the steak is resting, add the kale to the pan with a splash of water and let it wilt for a couple of minutes. Drain any residual water and add to the asparagus, mixing them together.

Slice the steak thinly and combine with the kale and asparagus. Spoon over the yogurt and lemon juice and add.

| PREP 5 minutes, plus 10 minutes resting | COOK 20 minutes | CALORIES 286 |
|---|---|---|

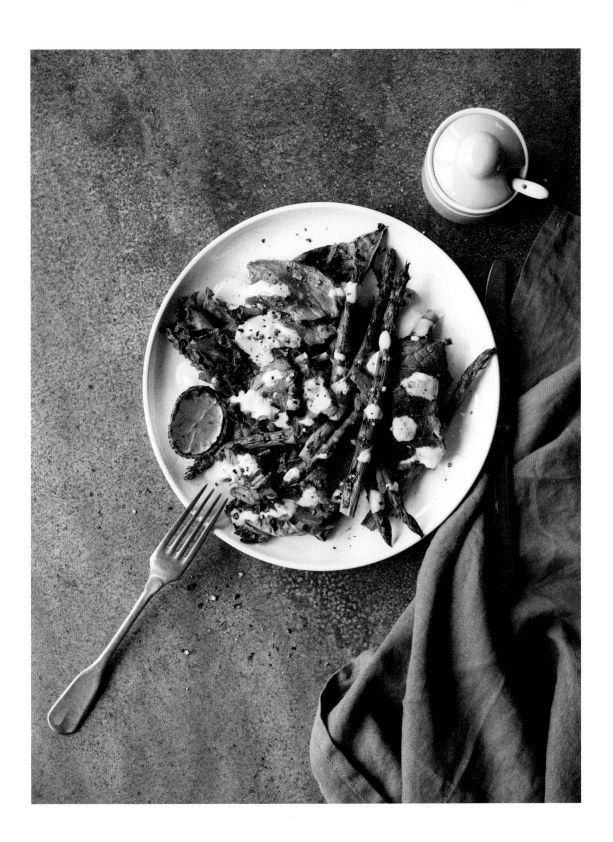

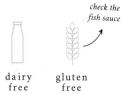

*check the fish sauce* ↗

dairy
free

gluten
free

# low-carb
# pad Thai

This is a healthy alternative to the traditional Thai favourite.
It contains plenty of fibre and nutrients from the vegetables,
and is satisfyingly filling while still being low in calories.
Once the ingredients have been prepped, it cooks in a flash.

*serves 2*

1 teaspoon sesame oil

1 egg, beaten

1 large garlic clove, crushed

2cm (1 inch) piece of fresh ginger,
   peeled and grated

1 red chilli, deseeded and
   thinly sliced

2 carrots, spiralised

2 courgettes, spiralised

40g (1½oz) bean sprouts

200g (7oz) raw peeled prawns

juice of 1 lime

1 tablespoon fish sauce

*to garnish*

a small handful of fresh coriander
   or Thai basil (about 10g/¼oz),
   torn or chopped

1 tablespoon chopped cashew nuts

Place a wok over a high heat and, when hot, add the
sesame oil.

Quickly stir-fry the egg, garlic, ginger and chilli, constantly
keeping things moving until the egg is scrambled (this will
literally be a matter of seconds, so keep an eye on it – things
can incinerate at speed in a wok).

Add the spiralised carrots and courgettes, and cook, stirring
constantly, for a minute or so.

Add the bean sprouts and prawns and cook for a further
2 minutes until the prawns have turned pale pink. Make
sure any liquid from the vegetables has cooked away.

Squeeze over the lime juice and add the fish sauce. Serve
immediately garnished with the coriander or Thai basil and
the cashew nuts.

| PREP 10 minutes | COOK 7 minutes | CALORIES 238 |
| --- | --- | --- |

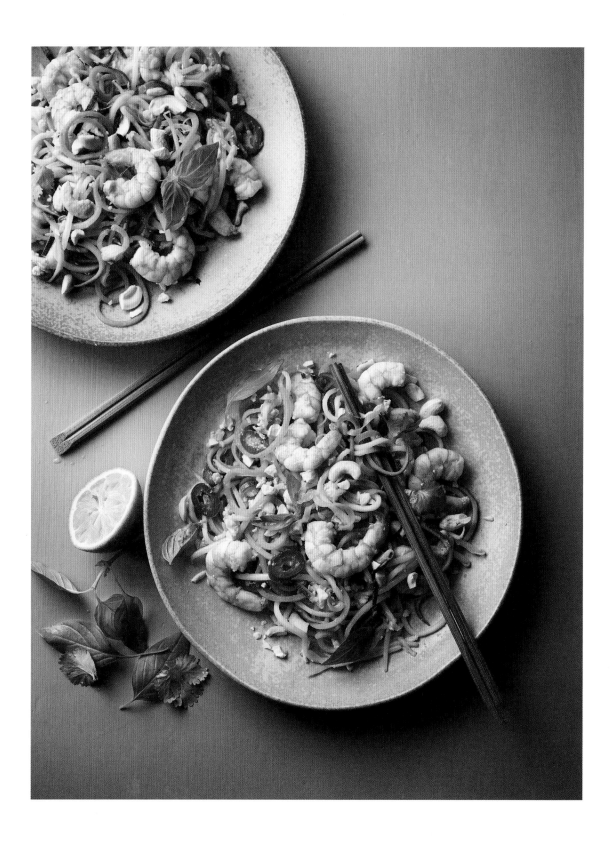

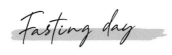

dairy
free

gluten
free

# bread-free burger with sauerkraut

*serves 2*

1 teaspoon sesame oil

2 teaspoons rapeseed oil

½ red onion, finely chopped

100g (3½oz) mushrooms
(button, chestnut, shiitake),
finely chopped

250g (9oz) minced beef (5% fat)
or turkey

2 teaspoons finely chopped
rosemary

1 gem lettuce, leaves separated

sea salt and freshly ground
black pepper

*to serve*

1 tablespoon sauerkraut (optional)

6 slices of cucumber

1 teaspoon tomato purée
per burger

With a few tweaks, it is possible to have something similar to a regular burger – except this one isn't drenched in fat and squashed between a carb-tastic bun. Any lean minced meat works for this recipe and adding a spoonful of sauerkraut is a great alternative for gherkin lovers, particularly as it helps maintain a healthy microbiome. Tomato purée is high in lycopene, a carotenoid antioxidant that supports healthy lungs, and is MUCH better for you than ketchup. Use liberally.

Heat half the oil in a frying pan over a medium heat. Add the onion, mushrooms and a splash of water, and cook for about 5 minutes, stirring occasionally, until they have softened. Set aside in a bowl until cool enough to handle.

Mix the minced beef or turkey and rosemary into the onion and mushrooms, seasoning well. Divide the mixture and shape into 2 burger patties about 2cm (¾ inch) thick.

Add the remaining oil to the pan over a medium-low heat and fry the burgers for about 10 minutes, turning every couple of minutes so they cook through.

Serve wrapped in the lettuce leaves and topped with the sauerkraut (if using), cucumber slices and tomato purée.

| PREP 5 minutes | COOK 20 minutes | CALORIES<br>216 (with minced beef)<br>205 (with minced turkey) |
|---|---|---|

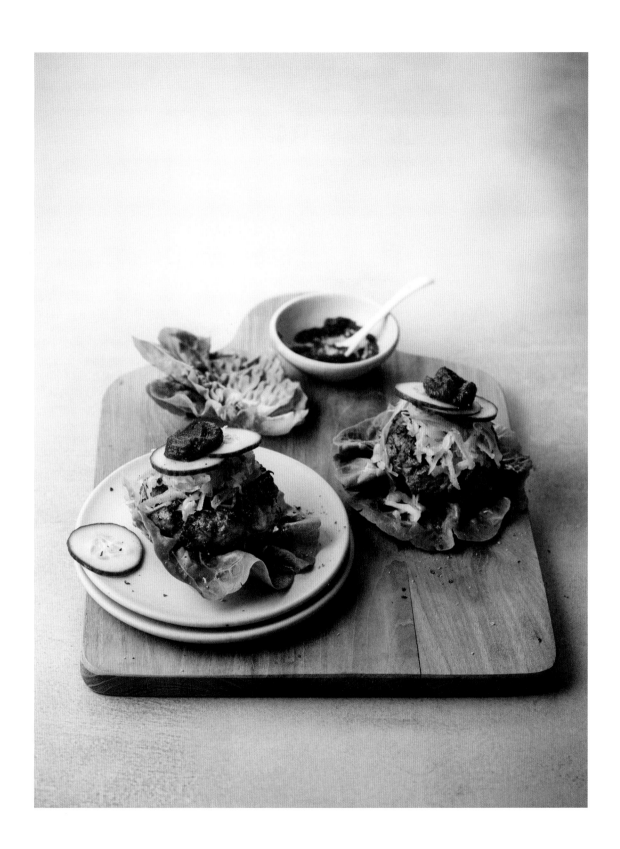

# chicken paillard

dairy
free

gluten
free

*serves 2*

2 organic or free-range chicken
  breasts (about 175g/6oz each)
sea salt and freshly ground
  black pepper
100g (3½oz) rocket or salad
  leaves, to serve

*for the marinade*

2 garlic cloves, grated
2 teaspoons picked thyme leaves
2 teaspoons finely chopped sage
juice of ½ lemon
1 tablespoon rapeseed oil

Chicken contains the amino acid tryptophan, which improves sleep and helps build muscle. It's really brought to life in this recipe by a delicious marinade of garlic, herbs and lemon. A helping of rocket on the side stimulates digestive enzymes with its bitterness.

Place the chicken breasts between two pieces of non-stick baking paper and bash with a meat tenderiser or rolling pin until about 5mm (¼ inch) thick. Place in a shallow dish.

Make the marinade by mixing the garlic, thyme, sage, lemon juice and rapeseed oil in a bowl. Pour it over the chicken, ensuring it is coated. Cover and leave to marinate in the fridge for a couple of hours.

Remove the chicken half an hour before cooking to bring it up to room temperature.

Heat a frying pan over a medium heat. Cook the chicken for about 2–3 minutes on each side, or until golden (there is oil in the marinade, so it shouldn't be necessary to add more).

Season well and serve with rocket or salad leaves on the side.

| PREP 10 minutes plus 2 hours marinating + 30 minutes resting | COOK 7 minutes | CALORIES 220 |
| --- | --- | --- |

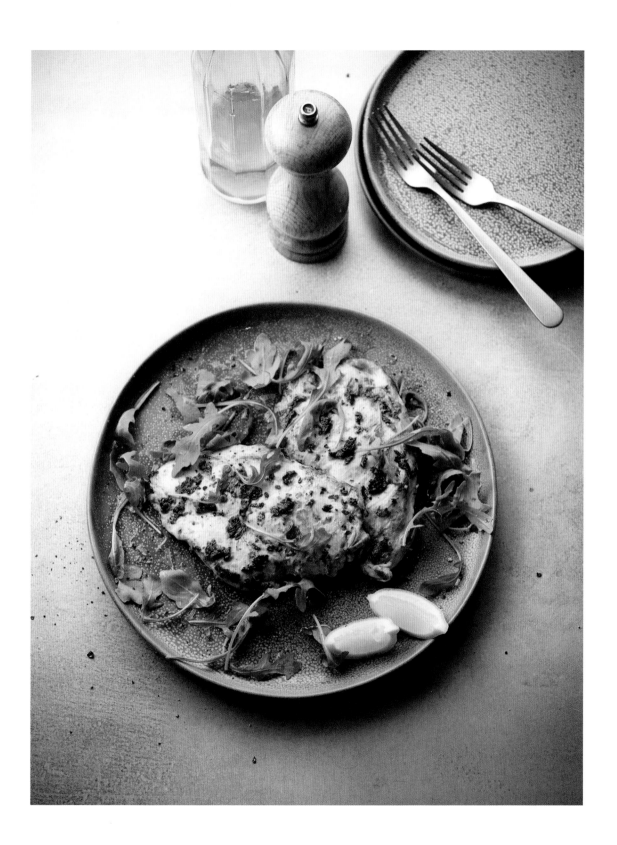

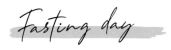

*Fasting day*

dairy
free

gluten
free

vegan

# vegan pancakes with chia seeds & agave

*serves 2 or 3*
(makes 6 pancakes)

100g (3½oz) buckwheat flour

1 teaspoon baking powder

220ml (8fl oz) almond milk

1 tablespoon chia seeds

2 teaspoons agave syrup

2 teaspoons coconut oil, at
   room temperature

pinch of salt

*to serve*

a handful of mixed berries
   of your choice

a squeeze of lemon juice

I know, I know. You're right. I AM spoiling you. These pancakes are gluten and dairy free and much healthier than their calorific cousins. They make a great weekend treat. A dollop of yogurt is a nice little addition of protein that works deliciously with the berries.

Mix the flour and baking powder together in a bowl. Add the nut milk, chia seeds, agave, half the coconut oil and the salt, then blend everything together thoroughly with an electric or hand whisk until the mixture is smooth and lump-free.

Melt the remaining coconut oil in a frying pan over a medium-high heat. Add a small ladle of the batter and let it spread a little. After a minute it should start to colour, so flip it over and cook the other side until golden. Set aside on a warmed plate and work through the rest of the batter.

Serve with your favourite mixed berries and a squeeze of lemon juice.

| PREP 5 minutes | COOK 15 minutes | CALORIES 279 for 2 and 186 for 3 |
| --- | --- | --- |

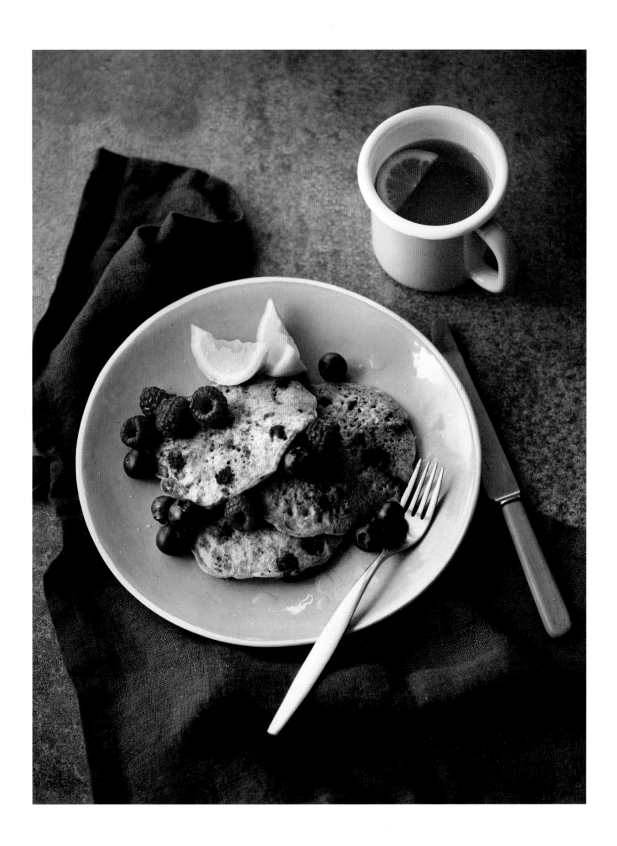

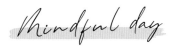
*mindful day*

dairy free · gluten free · vegan

# quinoa porridge with almonds & berries

*serves 1*

4 tablespoons quinoa
  (about 50g/1¾oz)
125ml (4fl oz) almond milk
100ml (3½fl oz) water
1 teaspoon ground cinnamon or
  nutmeg
½ tablespoon nut butter
  (almond or cashew)

*To serve*

a handful of mixed berries
  of your choice
1 tablespoon chopped
  almonds

Quinoa is a great alternative to oats and with the addition of the almonds, this porridge is a real protein hit. The berries give that extra boost of antioxidants and the little note of spice provides a perfect warming start to the day.

Put the quinoa, almond milk and water into a saucepan over a medium heat and bring to the boil. Reduce the heat to low and gently simmer for 15 minutes, giving it the occasional stir.

The quinoa should now be nice and soft, but not a mush. Stir in the cinnamon or nutmeg and the nut butter.

Serve with a handful of your favourite mixed berries and chopped almonds sprinkled over the top.

| PREP 5 minutes | COOK 17 minutes | CALORIES 280 |

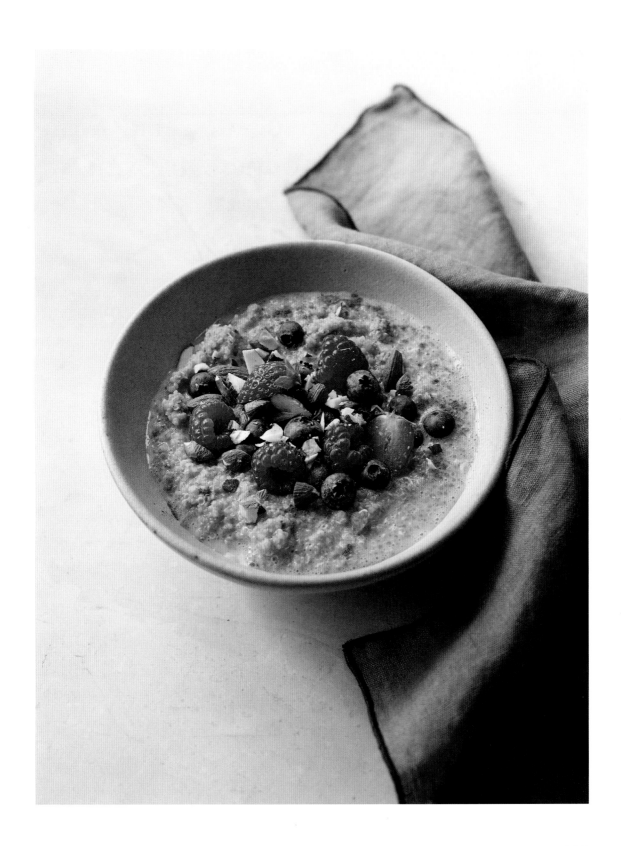

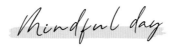

# egg & avocado salad with green goddess dressing

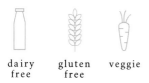

dairy free     gluten free     veggie

*serves 1*

30g (1¼oz) frozen edamame (soya) beans

½ avocado, sliced

6 radishes, sliced

1 teaspoon pumpkin or sunflower seeds

1 large egg

sea salt and freshly ground black pepper

*for the dressing*

large handful of spinach (80g/3oz)

a small handful of basil (about 15g/½oz)

a small handful of parsley (about 15g/½oz)

a small handful of fresh coriander (about 15g/½oz)

juice of 1 lime

2 teaspoons extra virgin olive oil

This is an absolute winner for breakfast, brunch or lunch. Eggs really are one of those any-time-of-day ingredients, with high levels of protein and B vitamins to keep you feeling full and energised. The herb-rich dressing is a superfood-loaded, immunity-boosting addition to liven up the party. It's best to use an egg at room temperature, as cold eggs straight from the fridge can crack as soon as they hit hot water.

Add the edamame to a saucepan of salted boiling water and cook for 3 minutes, when they should be al dente. Remove from the heat, drain and run them under cold water. Tip into a bowl. Remove the beans if still in their pods.

Add the avocado to the bowl, along with the radishes and pumpkin or sunflower seeds.

Put all the dressing ingredients into a blender and blitz until smooth. It should be fairly thick. Spoon half of it into the bowl with the chopped salad ingredients and mix until everything is coated.

Add the egg to a saucepan of boiling water and cook for 5½ minutes (this will give you a runny yolk, so cook it for a few more minutes if you prefer it a little firmer). Drain and run it under cold water so you can peel it without burning your fingers off. Cut it in half and place on top of the salad. Add a decent grind of salt and pepper before serving.

| PREP 5 minutes | COOK 15 minutes | CALORIES 382 |
| --- | --- | --- |

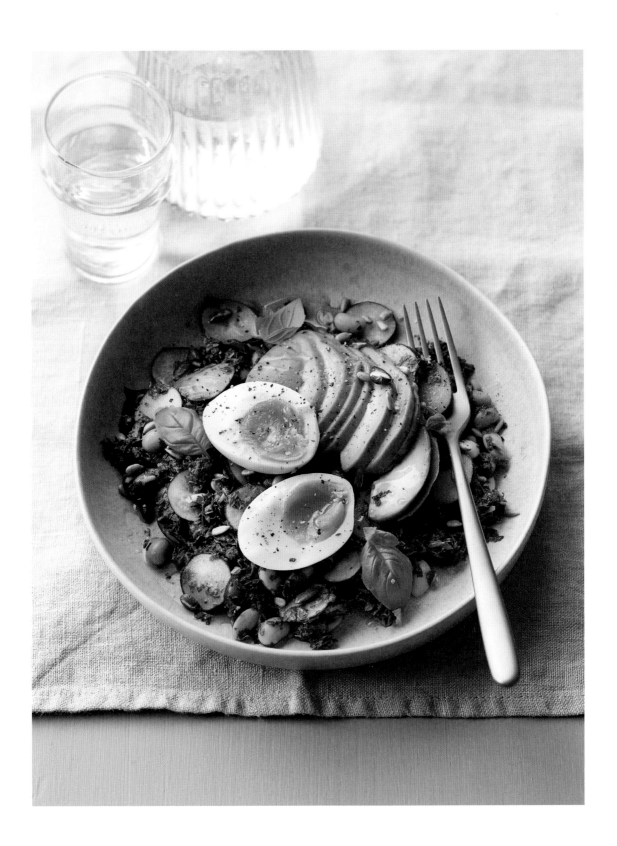

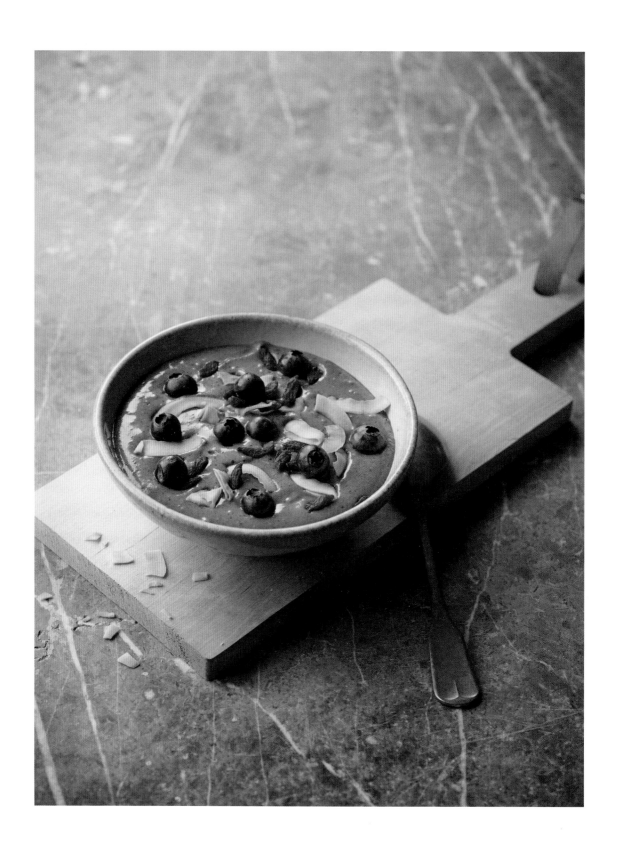

# morning smoothie bowl

dairy
free

gluten
free

vegan

This combination of antioxidant-rich berries and liver-loving greens means the day gets off to a nutrient-packed start. Avocado is a fantastic source of good fats and the protein powder keeps blood sugar levels perfectly balanced.

Blitz all the ingredients in a blender until smooth. If the mixture seems too thick, add a little water.

Spoon into a bowl and top with a small sprinkling of whatever you have to hand: sunflower and pumpkin seeds for a bit of crunch, goji berries and dried blueberries for a bit of chewiness or some coconut flakes.

## serves 1

¼ avocado (about 30g/1¼oz)

a handful of spinach or any other greens hanging around in the fridge (about 40g/1½oz), chopped

75g (2½oz) fresh or frozen mixed berries

2 tablespoons vegan protein powder (brown rice, pea or hemp), or 2 tablespoons nut yogurt (coconut, almond or cashew)

2 tablespoons berry powder (choose your favourite)

1 teaspoon coconut oil

1 tablespoon nut butter (almond, cashew, hazelnut)

250ml (9fl oz) your favourite nut milk

### to serve

2 tablespoons mixed berries

1 tablespoon sunflower and/or pumpkin seeds

a small handful of goji berries or dried blueberries

1 tablespoon coconut flakes

| PREP 5 minutes | CALORIES 255 |
| --- | --- |

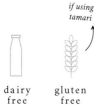

*if using tamari*

dairy
free

gluten
free

# golden chicken salad with sesame & ginger

## serves 1

1 tablespoon coconut oil

1 teaspoon ground turmeric

½ organic or free-range chicken
   breast (about 90g/3¼oz), sliced
   into strips 1cm (⅓ inch) thick

1 large carrot, thinly sliced
   or grated

½ courgette, thinly sliced or grated

½ white cabbage (about 50g/1¾oz),
   thinly sliced or grated

½ red pepper, cored, deseeded
   and thinly sliced

1 spring onion, thinly sliced

1½ teaspoons pumpkin seeds

sea salt and freshly ground
   black pepper

## for the dressing

2cm (1 inch) piece of fresh ginger,
   peeled and grated

1 small garlic clove, crushed

1 tablespoon apple cider vinegar

2 teaspoons sesame oil

1 tablespoon extra virgin olive oil

1 tablespoon tamari or soy sauce

juice of 1 lime

small pinch of chilli flakes

a small handful of mint (15g/½oz)

1½ teaspoons sunflower or
   pumpkin seeds

This Asian-inspired salad has plenty of nutrient-rich vegetables and protein-packed chicken, which works like a dream with the ginger and sesame. It's a good idea to make double the amount and keep half in the fridge, as it's delicious cold the next day.

Melt the coconut oil in a frying pan over a medium heat, stir in the turmeric, cook for 1 minute until fragrant, then add the chicken strips. Fry for about 6 minutes until lightly golden, making sure you turn them so they cook through. Season with salt and pepper and remove from the heat.

Put the carrot, courgette, cabbage, red pepper and spring onion into a salad bowl.

To make the dressing, place everything in a blender and blitz for about a minute. Don't worry if it looks a bit coarse and rustic. It's meant to.

Add the chicken to the salad and pour over the dressing. Toss well, then scatter over the seeds before serving.

| PREP 10 minutes | COOK 10 minutes | CALORIES 490 |
|---|---|---|

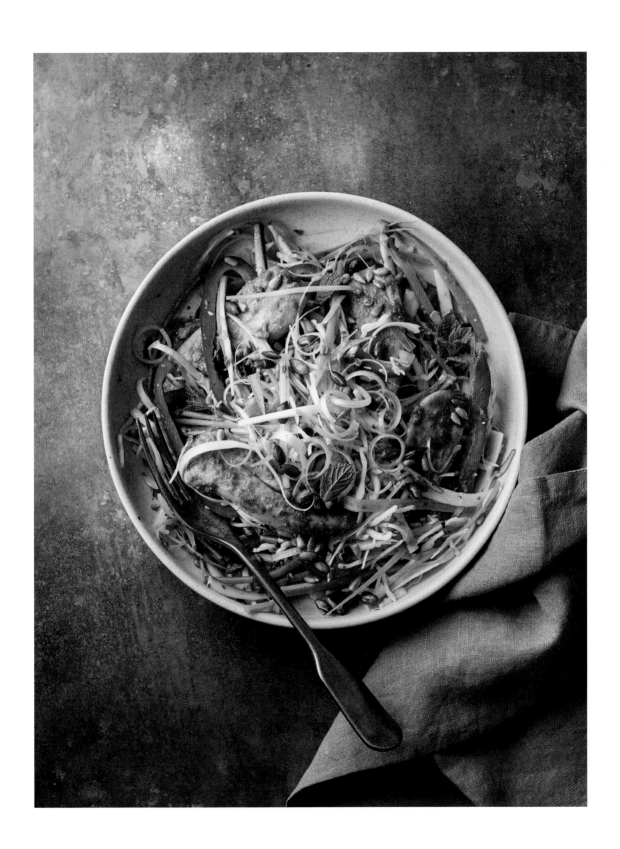

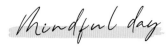

dairy
free

gluten
free

vegan

# chickpea, sweet potato & kale coconut curry

*serves 2*

2 teaspoons coconut oil

1 large shallot, finely chopped

2 large garlic cloves, grated

½ teaspoon ground turmeric

½ teaspoon ground cumin

2cm (1 inch) piece of fresh ginger, peeled and grated

½ teaspoon chilli flakes (this will make it medium spicy)

½ can (200g/7oz) of chopped tomatoes

1 sweet potato, cut into 1.5cm (½ inch) cubes

½ can (200g/7oz) of chickpeas, drained and rinsed

½ can (200ml/7fl oz) of light coconut milk

100g (3½oz) kale, stalks removed

a small handful of fresh coriander (15g/½oz), chopped

sea salt and freshly ground black pepper

This is what healthy comfort food looks like. It's a fantastic vegan alternative to the traditional Indian takeaway. The sweet potato promotes digestive health, as the soluble and insoluble fibre content supports a balanced microbiome. Serve with brown rice or quinoa and a squeeze of lime juice.

Melt the coconut oil in a large saucepan (preferably one with a lid) over a medium heat. Add the shallot and gently fry for a couple of minutes, or until soft.

Add the garlic, turmeric, cumin, ginger and chilli flakes and cook for a further minute until the garlic is lightly golden (make sure it doesn't catch).

Next, add the chopped tomatoes, sweet potato, chickpeas and coconut milk. Mix everything together well, cover with a lid and let it simmer away for about 20 minutes, or until you can easily pierce the sweet potato with the tip of a knife.

Stir in the kale and let it wilt – this should take 5 minutes. Season to taste, sprinkle over the coriander and serve.

| PREP 10 minutes | COOK 30 minutes | CALORIES 533 |
|---|---|---|

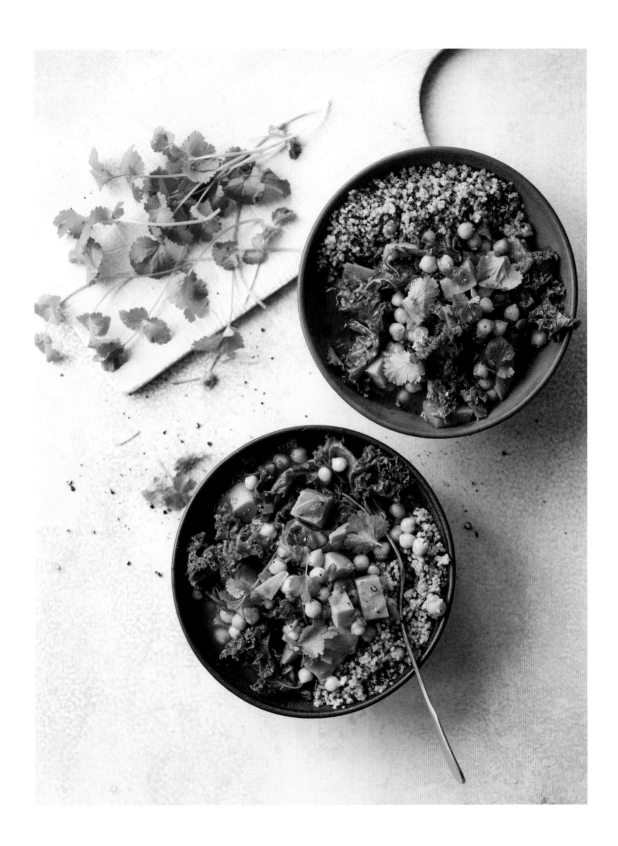

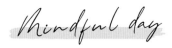

# broad beans, feta & chilli on toast

*veggie*

*serves 2*

150g (5½oz) fresh podded or frozen broad beans

20g (¾oz) feta

a small handful of rocket (about 15g/½oz)

1 garlic clove

1½ tablespoons extra virgin olive oil

juice of ½ lime

4 small slices of pumpernickel or rye bread, toasted

pinch of chilli flakes

sea salt and freshly ground black pepper

If toast for breakfast in the morning is a particular favourite, this recipe will appeal. Broad beans are a very rich source of fibre and B vitamins, so will energise you for the day. Salty feta is not only low in calories and fat, it contains beneficial bacteria and calcium, which is good for bone health. There's a lot to play with in this recipe – use edamame instead of broad beans if you prefer, or add an egg for a slightly more filling option.

Add the beans to a saucepan of salted boiling water and cook for 3 minutes. Remove from the heat, drain and run them under cold water until they're cool. If you're using fresh broad beans, remove each bean from its tough outer skin. Fiddly, but worth it.

Put half the beans, most of the feta, the rocket, garlic, oil and lime juice into a food processor and blend until smooth. Add the rest of the beans and briefly pulse until they are in chunky bits.

Spread the mixture onto the toast, season well, crumble over the rest of the feta and sprinkle over the chilli flakes.

| PREP 5 minutes | COOK 15 minutes | CALORIES 344 |
|---|---|---|

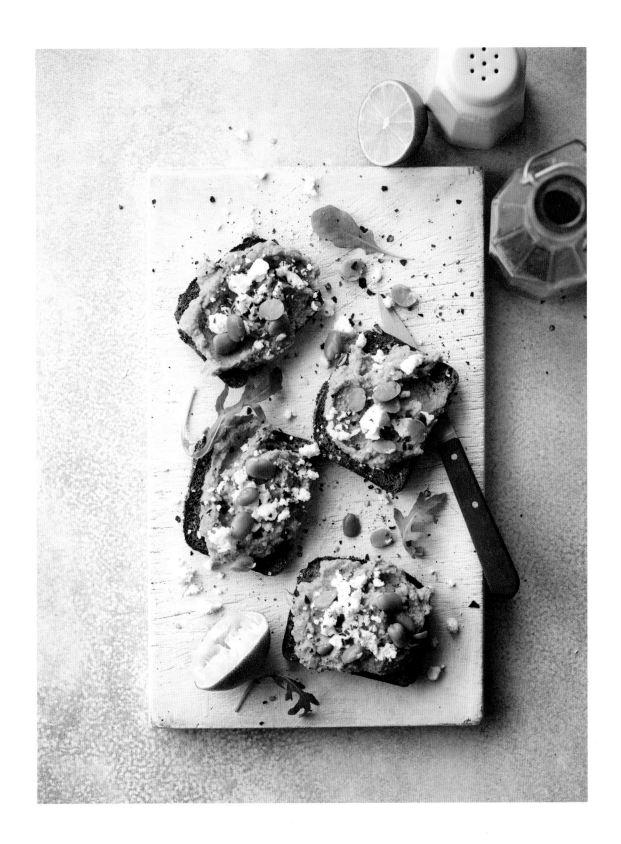

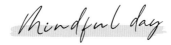
*Mindful day*

# Asian sea bass with tofu & kale broth

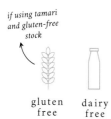

*if using tamari and gluten-free stock*

gluten
free

dairy
free

*serves 1*

1 tablespoon olive oil

a small handful of wild
  mushrooms (or any mushrooms
  of your choice), chopped

100g (3½oz) firm tofu, cubed

1 garlic clove, crushed or
  finely chopped

2cm (1 inch) piece of fresh
  ginger, peeled and grated

2 teaspoons tamari or soy sauce

200ml (7fl oz) vegetable stock
  (fresh, bouillon or cubes is fine)

100g (3½oz) kale, stalks removed

100g (3½oz) leafy greens (such as
  cabbage or chard)

1 sea bass fillet (about 180g/6oz),
  skin on

salt and freshly ground
  black pepper

Sea bass is a lovely, delicate white fish, which works perfectly with this nutrient-packed broth. Kale, cabbage and other greens are full of antioxidants, which help boost immunity. All this, and it's incredibly quick and easy to make for a light lunch or supper.

Place a saucepan over a medium heat and, when hot, add half the oil and gently fry the mushrooms, tofu, garlic and ginger for 2–3 minutes. Add a splash of water if necessary.

Add the tamari or soy sauce and vegetable stock, bring to the boil, then reduce the heat and simmer for a further couple of minutes. Add the kale and leafy greens.

Lightly season the sea bass with salt and pepper. Heat the remaining oil in a frying pan over a medium heat. When hot, add the sea bass, skin side down, and cook for a couple of minutes, or until the skin is golden and crispy. Reduce the heat a little, then flip the fish over and cook for a further minute or so.

Pour the broth into a warmed bowl and place the sea bass on top to serve.

| PREP 10 minutes | COOK 15 minutes | CALORIES 427 |
|---|---|---|

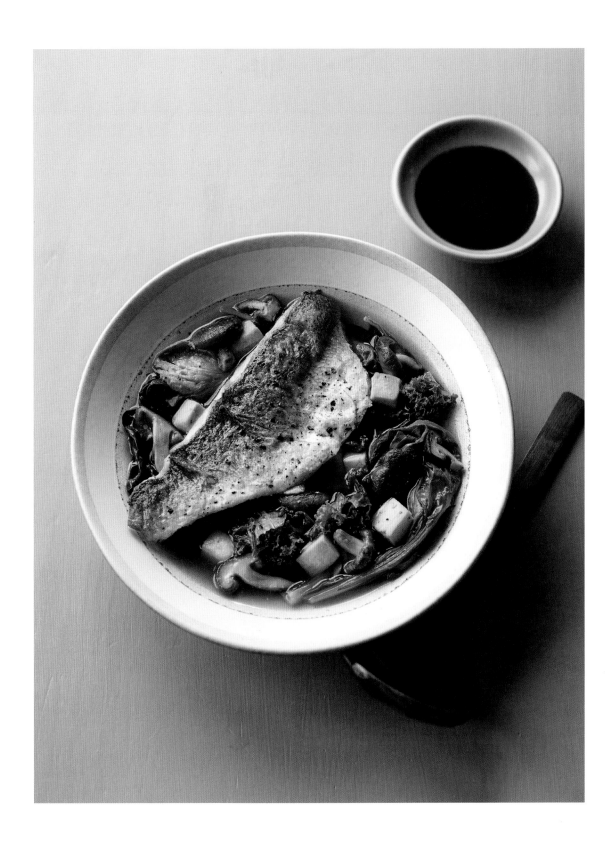

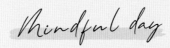

# crunchy tabbouleh with turkey & tahini dressing

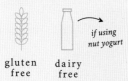

gluten
free

dairy
free

*if using
nut yogurt*

*serves 2*

100g (3½oz) precooked quinoa

100g (3½oz) cherry tomatoes,
   quartered

¼ cucumber, cut into small cubes

¼ red onion, finely chopped

a small handful of parsley (about
   15g/½oz), chopped

a small handful of mixed seeds
   (pumpkin, sunflower)

1 tablespoon extra virgin olive oil

juice of ½ lemon

2 turkey breasts (about 125g/4½oz
   each), sliced into strips 1cm
   (½ inch) thick

1 teaspoon rapeseed oil

sea salt and freshly ground
   black pepper

*for the dressing*

1 tablespoon tahini paste

1 tablespoon natural live or
   almond/coconut yogurt

½ teaspoon agave syrup

½ garlic clove

a squeeze of lemon juice

3 tablespoons water

This is a take on the glorious Middle Eastern salad. Adding seeds gives it a delicious nutrient-filled crunch, while the turkey is low in fat and an excellent source of tryptophan. The protein-rich dressing of tahini and yogurt brings the whole thing together like a dream.

Put the quinoa, tomatoes, cucumber, onion, parsley, seeds, oil and lemon juice into a bowl and mix everything together well. Season to taste.

Toss the sliced turkey in rapeseed oil and season. Heat a frying pan over a medium heat and fry the turkey for about 6 minutes, or until golden and cooked through.

In a bowl, mix all the dressing ingredients together. Plate up with the quinoa and vegetable mix first, followed by the turkey and finally pour over the dressing.

| PREP 1 minute | COOK 10 minutes | CALORIES 360 |
| --- | --- | --- |

# red rice risotto & cavolo nero

if using
gluten-free
stock

if using
veg stock

gluten
free

veggie

serves 2

The red colour of the rice comes from the anthocyanins, a type of flavonoid antioxidant. Red rice is also packed with B vitamins and is considerably higher in fibre than white rice. I love immune-boosting cavolo nero, but any dark leafy greens would be delicious here. Wild mushrooms contain selenium, another powerful antioxidant. In fact, I'm not sure how much healthier this recipe could actually be.

Heat the oil in a large saucepan over a medium heat and then add the onion and fry for 5 minutes until softened. The garlic goes in next for a further minute, followed by the mushrooms for 3 minutes until softened.

Drain the rice and add to the pan, stirring everything together well before adding the stock. Bring to the boil and then reduce to a simmer for about 25 minutes, stirring occasionally until almost all the water has been absorbed and the rice has a creamy consistency. Add the cavolo nero, stir well and then add the spinach. Let them wilt in the heat for about 3 minutes.

Season to taste and serve sprinkled with cheese on top.

1 tablespoon olive oil

1 red onion, finely chopped

2 garlic cloves, chopped

100g (3½oz) wild mushrooms (shiitake, girolle, oyster), thinly sliced

85g (3oz) red rice, covered with water and soaked overnight, or for at least 2 hours before cooking

250ml (9fl oz) organic chicken or vegetable stock (fresh, bouillon or cubes is fine)

50g (1¾oz) cavolo nero (or any dark leafy green, such as kale), sliced

50g (1¾oz) spinach, chopped

sea salt and freshly ground black pepper

50g (1¾oz) Parmesan cheese, to serve (or choose a vegan option)

| PREP 10 minutes plus soaking time | COOK 40 minutes | CALORIES 283 |
| --- | --- | --- |

*if using
corn tortillas*

gluten
free

# cheat's pizza

serves *2*

2 medium wholewheat flour or
   corn tortillas

2 heaped tablespoons tomato purée

1 garlic clove, grated

125g (4½oz) mozzarella, torn into
   small chunks

4 slices of Parma ham, fat
   removed and torn into bits

6 sun-dried tomatoes, roughly
   chopped

a small handful of basil
   (about 15g/½oz)

½ teaspoon chilli flakes (optional)

85g (3oz) rocket

2–3 teaspoons olive oil,
   for drizzling

sea salt and freshly ground
   black pepper

I love pizza. I can't imagine living without it – so I've decided not to. These are a healthier, lighter version that are quick and convenient to make. I keep a stack of tortilla wraps in my freezer at all times, which means these can be made on the spur of the moment. Kids love them too and it's easy to load them up with any vegetables, as well as the odd slice of ham. Mindful does not have to be a complete departure from all our favourite foods. It just means getting inventive.

Preheat the oven to 240°C (475°F), gas mark 9. Line a baking tray with non-stick baking paper.

Place the tortillas on the lined tray. Spread the tomato purée over the tortillas, almost to the edge but leaving a small border. Evenly scatter over the garlic, mozzarella, Parma ham, sun-dried tomatoes and basil.

Place in the oven for around 6 minutes, or until the mozzarella has melted.

Remove from the oven, scatter over the chilli flakes (if using) and the rocket and drizzle over the oil. Season well before serving.

| PREP 5 minutes | COOK 10 minutes | CALORIES |
|---|---|---|
| | | 406 (corn tortillas) 451 (wholewheat) |

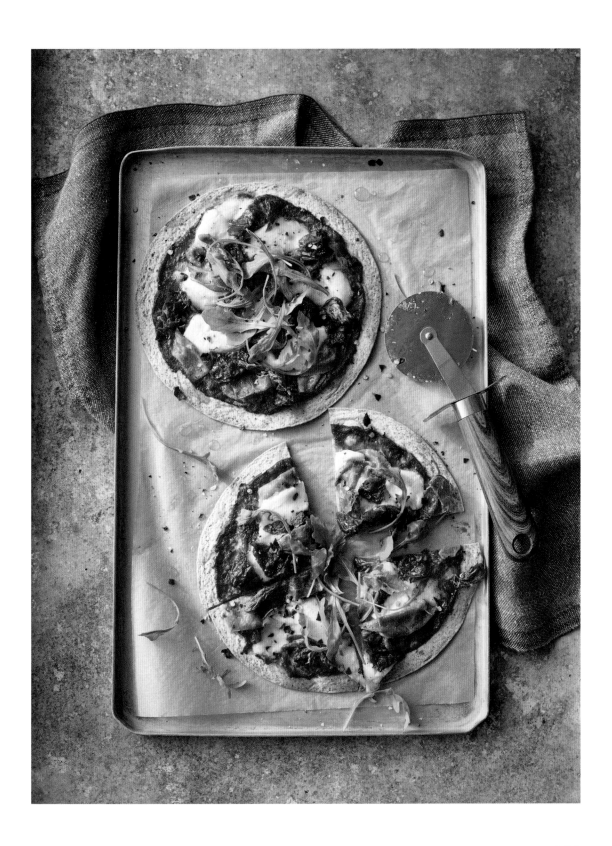

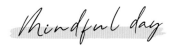

dairy free    gluten free    vegan

# roasted beetroot & spinach curry

serves 2

3 beetroots (about 500g/1lb 2oz), cut into thinnish wedges

1 tablespoon rapeseed oil

2 shallots, finely chopped

3 garlic cloves, grated

2cm (1 inch) piece of fresh ginger, peeled and grated

1 teaspoon agave syrup

½ teaspoon ground turmeric

½ teaspoon ground cumin

2 tablespoons finely chopped cashews

1 red chilli, deseeded and thinly sliced

400ml (14fl oz) can of light coconut milk or coconut drink

400g (14oz) can of chickpeas, drained and rinsed

200g (7oz) spinach, chopped

1 tablespoon chopped fresh coriander

juice of 1 lime

½ tablespoon pine nuts

sea salt and freshly ground black pepper

Beetroot is overflowing with nutrients, such as folate and vitamin C, and is a great source of fibre. Combined with iron-rich spinach, this vivid-red, rustic dish is just the ticket for a cosy night on the sofa. (Just make sure you don't spill it because it won't be coming out any time soon. Thanks to my very small son for this important lesson.) Serve with brown rice, quinoa or rye bread.

Preheat the oven to 200°C (400°F), gas mark 6.

Place the beetroots in a roasting tin, sprinkle with a pinch of salt and roast for 20 minutes.

While they are cooking, heat the rapeseed oil in a large saucepan over a medium heat. Cook the shallots for about 5 minutes until softened, then add the garlic, ginger, agave, turmeric, cumin, nuts and chilli and cook for a further couple of minutes.

Pour in the coconut milk and bring up to a simmer for 10 minutes. Add the chickpeas and beetroots and simmer for a further 5 minutes.

Stir in the spinach until it wilts (this will literally take a minute or so), followed by the coriander. Squeeze in the lime juice, sprinkle over the pine nuts and season to taste.

| PREP 10 minutes | COOK 30 minutes | CALORIES 631 |
|---|---|---|

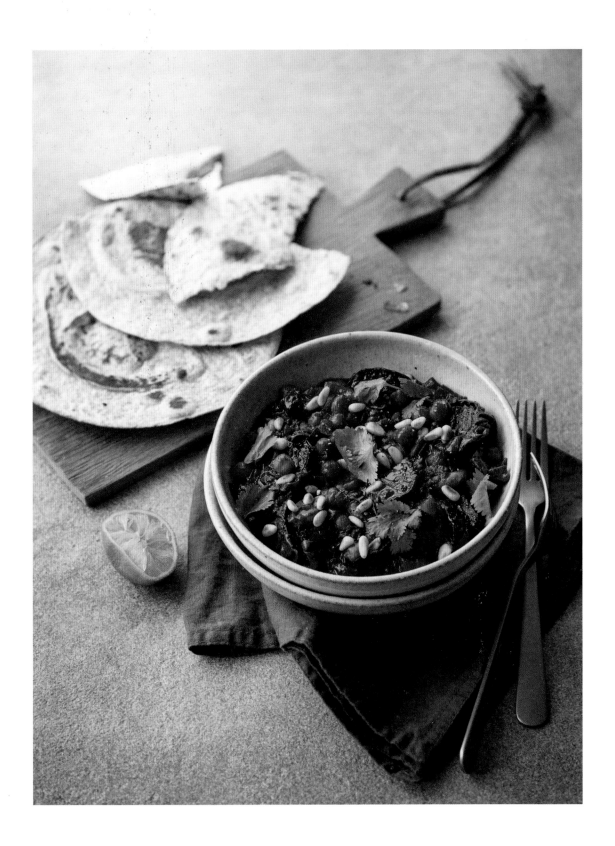

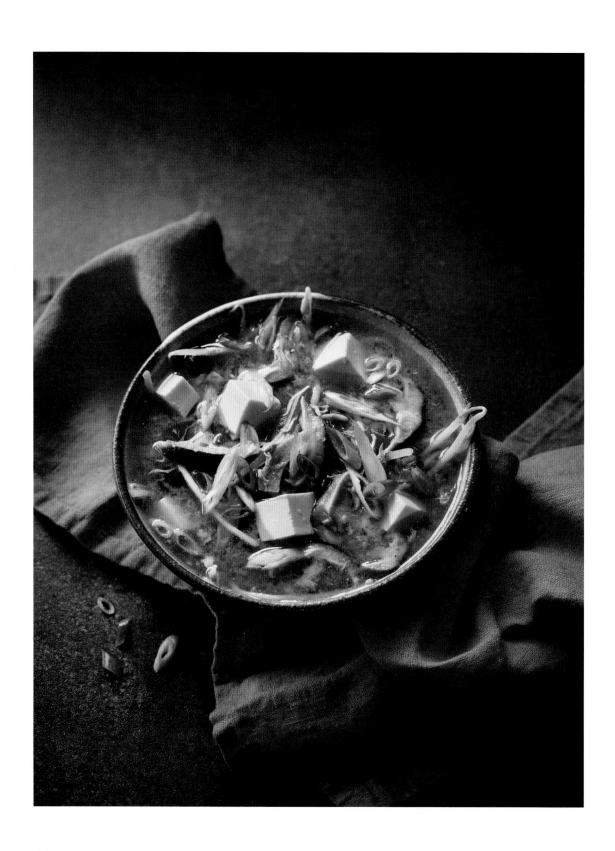

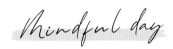

# hearty hot
# & sour soup

if using tamari
and gluten-free
stock

dairy
free

gluten
free

veggie

if using tofu
and veg stock

Warming and delicious, this spicy soup is based on the Asian classic and is packed with flavour. The light, crunchy bean sprouts can improve blood lipid levels, which your heart will love you for. The egg and chicken both provide protein, but it's easy to make this recipe vegetarian by using tofu and vegetable stock instead.

Heat the oil in a saucepan over a medium heat and then add the chilli, garlic and ginger and cook, stirring for 1 minute. Next add the mushrooms and gently fry for about 3 minutes, or until softened.

Add the tamari or soy, rice wine vinegar, agave and stock. Bring to the boil and then reduce to a simmer for 10 minutes, when the soup should be slightly reduced. Add the bean sprouts and chicken or tofu and stir well for a couple of minutes to ensure they're warmed through.

Crack in the egg, mixing quickly so that it scrambles but breaks up in the heat.

Serve in bowls with the spring onions sprinkled over the top and a squeeze of lime juice.

*serves 2*

1 tablespoon rapeseed oil

1 red chilli, deseeded and cut into strips

1 garlic clove, grated

2cm (1 inch) piece of fresh ginger, peeled and grated

130g (4½oz) shiitake mushrooms, sliced

1 tablespoon tamari or soy sauce

2 tablespoons rice wine vinegar

1 teaspoon agave syrup

750ml (1⅓ pint) organic chicken or vegetable stock (fresh, bouillon or cubes is fine)

100g (3½oz) bean sprouts

70g (2½oz) leftover chicken, shredded, or firm tofu, cubed

1 large organic or free-range egg

sea salt and freshly ground black pepper

*to serve*

1 spring onion, thinly sliced

juice of ½ lime

| PREP 5 minutes | COOK 25 minutes | CALORIES<br>231 (with chicken)<br>193 (with tofu) |
|---|---|---|

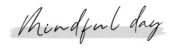

  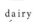

gluten
free

dairy
free

# salmon & kale salad with chickpea croutons

## serves 2

½ can (200g/7oz) of chickpeas, drained and rinsed

1 tablespoon olive oil

1 teaspoon garlic powder

½ red onion, thinly sliced

juice of ½ lime

40g (1½oz) tempeh, cut into small cubes

1 salmon fillet (about 125g/ 4½oz), skin on

120g (4½oz) kale, stalks removed

sea salt and freshly ground pepper

## for the dressing

15g (½oz) cashew nuts, soaked overnight (leave in the refrigerator in a bowl of water)

1 teaspoon Dijon mustard

1 teaspoon olive oil

½ garlic clove

juice of ½ lemon

1 tablespoon water

Packed with omega-3, protein, B vitamins and selenium, salmon is a wonder fish. Chickpeas are a great source of fibre and make a delicious snack when roasted and crunchy; I recommend finishing them off with a little salt and some apple cider vinegar.

Preheat the oven to 200°C (400°F), gas mark 6. Pat the chickpeas dry with kitchen paper, so they crisp up when they're roasted. Tip them into a shallow roasting tin, pour over half the oil, add the garlic powder and mix everything together. Season well. Roast for about 20 minutes, or until crispy. Remove from the oven and allow to cool a little.

Meanwhile, place the onion in a small bowl, squeeze over the lime juice and leave to pickle.

Heat the rest of the oil in a frying pan over a medium heat and fry the tempeh and the salmon, skin side down, for 2 minutes before turning over and frying for 2 more minutes, or until cooked through. The tempeh should be lightly browned on all sides. Season and set aside to cool. Remove the skin from the salmon (be sure to eat it as a snack) and flake the flesh.

Put all the dressing ingredients into a blender and blitz until creamy and smooth, adding a little water to thin if necessary. Place the kale in a bowl, pour over half the dressing and toss. Add the salmon, tempeh, chickpeas and pickled onions, then drizzle the dressing over the top. Season well before serving.

| PREP 5 minutes plus soaking time | COOK 30 minutes | CALORIES 406 |
| --- | --- | --- |

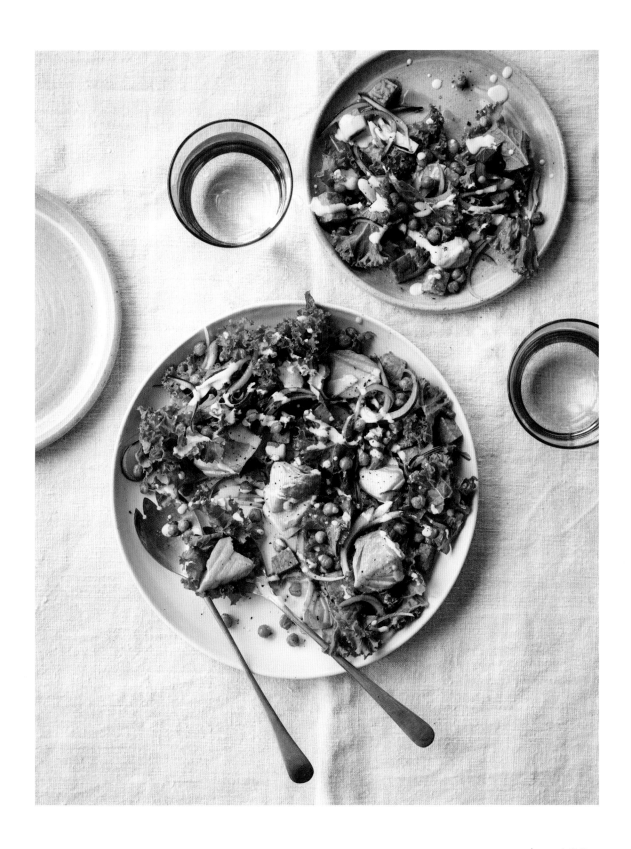

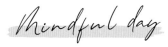 

# prawn & avocado summer rolls

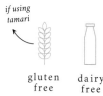

*if using tamari*

gluten free    dairy free

*serves 2* (makes 6 rolls)

130g (4½oz) red or white cabbage, thinly sliced

1 carrot, grated

1 tablespoon lime juice

½ tablespoon sesame oil

6 rice papers (22cm/8½ inches) in diameter)

12 mint leaves

12 cooked, peeled king prawns

½ avocado, cut into 6 slices

sea salt and freshly ground black pepper

*for the tahini dipping sauce*

3 tablespoons tahini paste

1 tablespoon sesame oil

3 tablespoons water

1 small garlic clove, grated

1cm (⅓ inch) piece of fresh ginger, peeled and grated

2 tablespoons lime juice

2 tablespoons rice wine vinegar

1 teaspoon agave syrup

1 teaspoon tamari or soy sauce

pinch of chilli flakes

These fresh, vibrant rolls have an Asian note to them, especially with the dipping sauce, which is full of flavour. With plenty of fibre and texture, they not only look beautiful, but are hugely versatile – from a light lunch, to a snack, to a canapé. Take your pick.

Put the cabbage and carrot into a bowl, mix in the lime juice and sesame oil, then season.

Make the dipping sauce by mixing the tahini, sesame oil and water together in a bowl until the tahini has thinned out. Add the garlic, ginger, lime juice, rice vinegar, agave and tamari or soy. Sprinkle with the chilli flakes.

Fill a shallow dish with water and soak the first rice paper for about 20 seconds until it's soft enough to use. Place it on a flat surface. Spoon some of the cabbage mixture along the centre of the rice paper, then add 2 mint leaves, 2 prawns and a slice of avocado. Fold the edge of the paper nearest to you over the filling, then roll it away from you so the filling is tightly wrapped (the rice paper should be quite sticky by now). Fold each end in. Repeat this process until all 6 are complete.

Serve with the tahini sauce for dipping.

| PREP 15 minutes | CALORIES 472 |
|---|---|

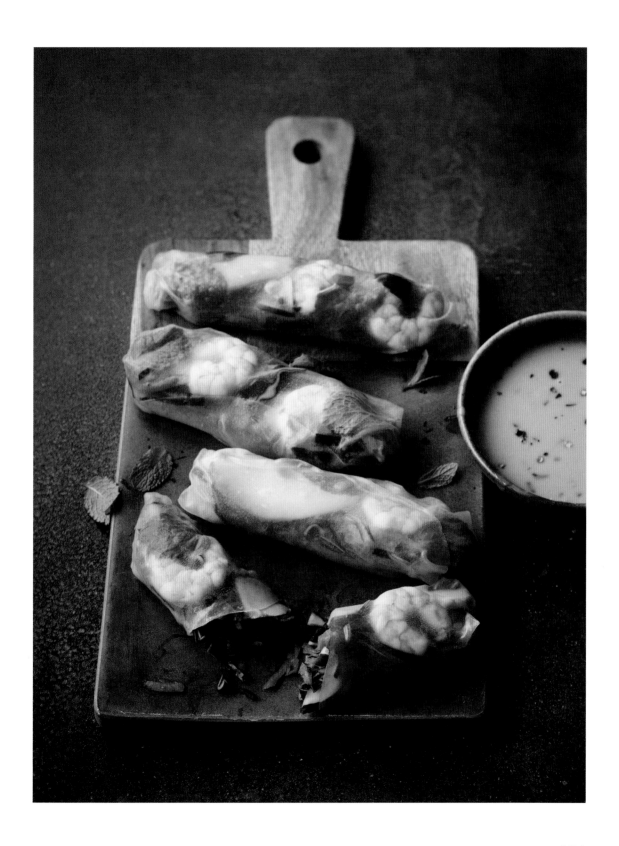

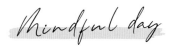

gluten
free

dairy
free

# flourless chocolate
# chip cookies

*serves* 6 (makes 12 cookies)

1 egg

75g (2½oz) coconut sugar

100g (3½oz) coconut oil, melted

90g (3¼oz) rolled oats

150g (5½oz) ground nuts (almonds, cashews, hazelnuts)

1 tablespoon finely chopped nuts (almonds, cashews, hazelnuts, walnuts, macadamia)

pinch of ground cinnamon

pinch of salt

100g (3½oz) plain dark chocolate (minimum 70% cocoa), chopped

Sticky and delicious, these cookies are a healthier alternative to their badly behaved shop-bought relations. Refined sugars are processed and have no nutritional value, while natural sugars, like the coconut variety we're using here, contain a fibre called inulin. It's not completely saintly, but it has a lower glycaemic index, which makes it a little gentler on blood sugar levels. In combination with the oats, which are really high in fibre, these gluten-free cookies won't cause a wild blood sugar spike.

Preheat the oven to 180°C (350°F), gas mark 4. Line a baking tray with non-stick baking paper.

Mix all the ingredients together in a bowl and then spoon the mixture onto the lined baking tray. Make sure each spoonful is well spaced out and flatten them down a bit so they resemble a cookie shape. How many cookies the mixture makes will depend on how big you want them – I usually make around 12, but they're not perfect and nor should they be. Press each one down a little. Bake in the oven for 10 minutes and leave to cool on a wire rack.

They'll keep for a week in an airtight container.

| PREP 10 minutes | COOK 10 minutes | CALORIES 260 |
| --- | --- | --- |

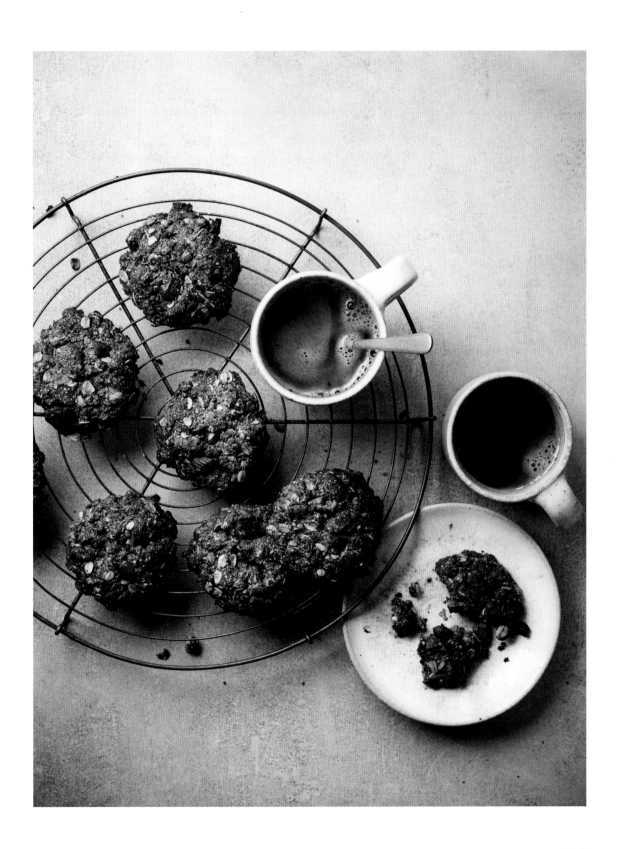

# supplement codes

It may be screamingly obvious by now that I am ALL about the wonder of supplements and so I have developed my own range, based on potent combinations of high-quality ingredients that I know deliver amazing results. To make this really easy for you, we have included super high-tech codes below which will take you straight to the relevant website page for the supplement programmes that specially align with the goals you want to achieve.

## HOW TO SCAN:
▶ Open the camera app on your smartphone.
▶ Hold it over the image of the code.
▶ A link will appear at the top of your screen.
▶ Find the supplements of your dreams waiting for you.

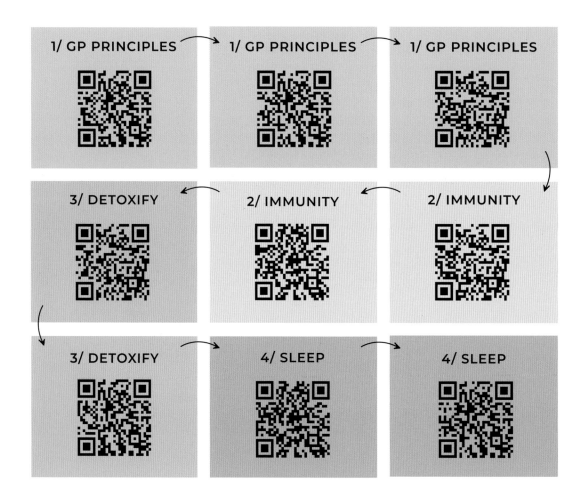

# index

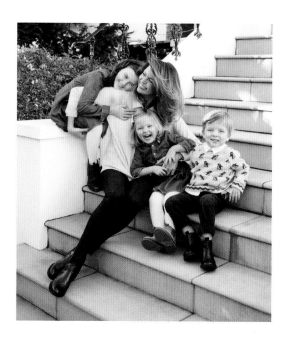

# acknowledgements

To my family, who had to tolerate my being locked away in a room for most of 2020 – I love you very much. I'm hoping that my twins, Iris and Caspar, are too young to remember how I told them that they weren't allowed to see Mummy for the whole of the winter. To my eldest, Maia – thank you for letting me lie on your yoga mat, surrounded by tortoises, and cry over the Krebs cycle. And to my husband, David. I originally wrote that I loved turmeric honey on toast more than you, but it got cut. Obviously, I didn't mean it. And my parents – who have tirelessly supported me, even when I probably didn't deserve it. You are all endlessly patient and I'm very grateful.

Clare Bennett, my brilliant and talented writer and friend. I can't imagine this project having happened without you. You have been so incredibly supportive throughout this journey; I loved every moment of working with you, and I am so very proud of what we have created.

To my agent, the fabulous Adrian Sington – thank you for your guidance and for believing in this book from start to finish. Huge thanks to Louise McKeever, Judith Hannam, Nikki Dupin,

Sophie Elletson and all the team at Kyle for all your hard work and for helping make this book happen. Enormous thanks to my friend, the amazingly talented Kate Martin for the lovely photos of my family and me. And to Kate Whittaker, who took such great photos of the recipes in this book.

Thanks to all the friends who have championed and supported me tirelessly through the madness of writing a book during lockdown. I couldn't appreciate you all more. Special thanks to Celia Walden, who so sweetly and generously spent hours with me thinking of book ideas over very important work martinis in the Electric.

The fantastic GP Nutrition team – thank you for everything. And to Jennifer Martin and Jo Lewin for your dedicated research skills.

And to my clients – you have all helped me become a better nutritionist with your stories and journeys. You have each informed my understanding of the personal side of nutrition, which has in turn shaped the nature of this book. My hope is that this will in turn help others.